osmetic Chemistry

r the skin treatment therapist

Florence Barrett-Hill

Proudly published by
Virtual Beauty Corporation Ltd.
P.O. Box 322 Whangaparaoa
New Zealand 0943

Cosmetic Chemistry

By Florence Barrett-Hill

Designed & printed in New Zealand

National library of New Zealand Cataloguing Publication Data
Barrett-Hill, Florence.
Cosmetic Chemistry
1st edition.
Includes bibliographical references and glossary
ISBN 978-0-473-12467-0 (soft cover)

NOTICE TO THE READER

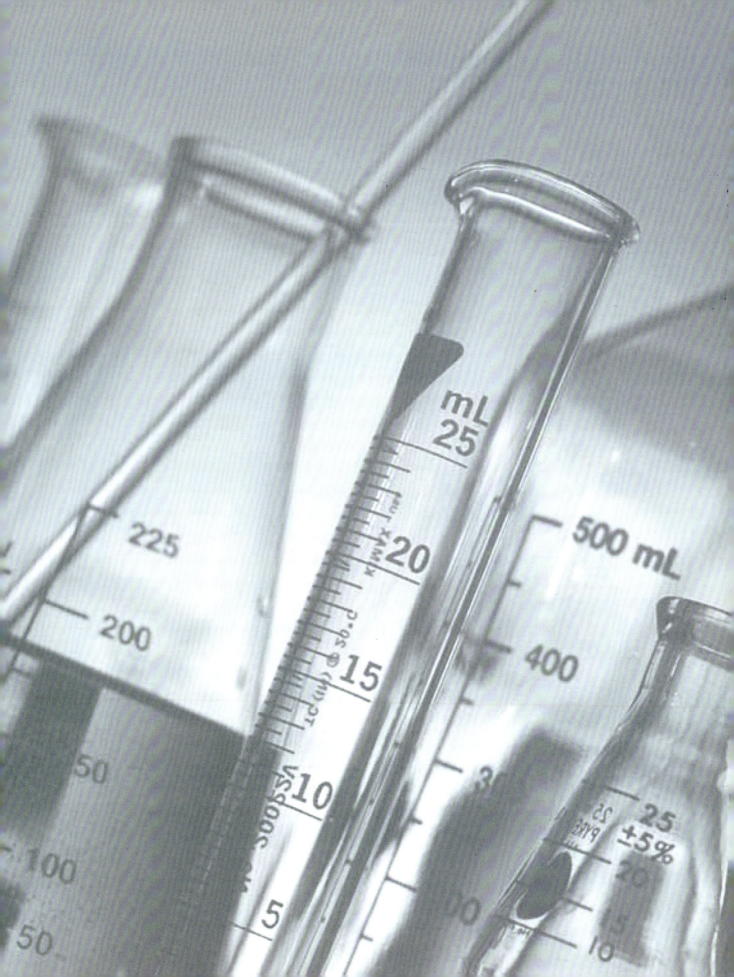

Contents

Chapter one: Understanding formulations

Chapter one: Understanding formulations

Welcome back..

I hope you have all experienced a degree of success from practising the techniques and applying the information shared in my previous book, Advanced Skin Analysis.
There is still more knowledge that will make a difference to diagnosing and treating your client's skin, and much of this comes in understanding a little basic cosmetic chemistry.

Correct skin analysis is only part of being a successful skin treatment therapist correct choice of treatment modality comes next. Along with that choice must come the correct range of chemicals/actives the damaged cells and systems will require for repair and maintenance.
The correct and appropriate choice will ultimately result in a correct procedure that will fulfil both you and your clients' expectations.

It is not however, only being able to write a treatment program. This book will also help you choose a new skin care line for clinical use. How to make that correct choice is once again dependant on comprehensive knowledge of the skins cells and supporting systems. This knowledge you would have gained from reading my first book, which I will often refer back to in this manuscript. I will do this to ensure that you truly understand the cells and systems that create that wonderful system the skin.

Cosmetic chemistry is not a difficult subject to comprehend once you understand what stimulus and nourishment skin cells and their ecosystems require to function correctly and efficiently.
Equally important in cosmetic chemistry is to be aware of chemicals and substances that may cause adverse effects on skin cells and systems under certain circumstances and know to avoid.

The first chapter is a basic " what is in a formulation introduction" and in chapters two through four, I will be presenting the information in the same format of categorising skin conditions by their respective characters of Texture, Colour and Secretion that is used for an advanced skin analysis.

So special thanks go to my husband Ralph for his unwavering support and belief, not to mention the fantastic graphics throughout the book that he created for me. I would like to thank my mentors, peers and colleagues around the world that took the time out to proof read and offer feedback regarding content, with special mentions to Anne Barnes and Reika Roberts from Australia, Alexandra J. Zani from the U.S., Dr Lance Setterfield and René Serbon from Canada, and Ruth Minoletti, Nicki Caro and Donna Gershinson from the U.K.. All of your input was invaluable and I am privileged to know you all. To all of you who provided input, opinion and support, Ralph and I thank you all very much.

Enjoy expanding the horizons of your chosen profession. It will reward you with achievement, confidence and respect.

Warm Regards

Florence

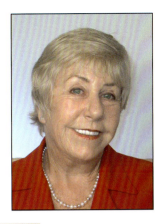

About the author

New Zealand born Florence Barrett-Hill is one of the world's leading independent technical educators in the field of professional skin treatment therapies and dermal science with over 30 years of experience in all aspects of professional beauty therapy and paramedical skin care to share.

From a background in pharmacy, and later skin treatment therapy, CIDESCO and ITEC qualified Florence has experience from operating specialist clinics, through to paramedical experience in the post operative care of burns survivors and plastic surgery patients. Florence is also a researcher, author, and trainer of both generic and brand specific philosophies and understands the wide range of treatment modalities and their place in the industry.
Florence intimately knows her subject and is passionate about continually raising the standards of professional skin care to meet new markets.

Florence is the creator of the internationally recognised Pastiche Method of advanced skin analysis that has been taught in it's many evolving forms globally since 1994, with thousands of beauty and skin treatment therapists from around the world taking their careers to the next level from the training.
The popular training course is the core of Florence's first book, (and the prelude to this manuscript) Advanced Skin Analysis, (ISBN 978-0-476-00665-2) first published in 2004. This ground breaking book continues to receive critical acclaim across the professional beauty and skin care industry globally with thousands of copies sold along with translations in to four languages.

Florence is a sought after presenter of technical matters pertaining to skin treatment therapy, and travels internationally sharing her knowledge with individuals and groups who believe the future of professional skin care lies with a scientific foundation.
Many leading icons in professional skin care recognise Florence as one of the few people uniquely capable to take professional skin treatment therapy and non-invasive aesthetic medicine in to the realms of scientific skin care, and her expertise is sought by organisations internationally.

Other titles by Florence Barrett-Hill:

Advanced Skin Analysis ISBN 978-0-476-00665-2
The Aesthetic Clinicians Dictionary ISBN 978-0-473-15964-1
The Aesthetic Clinicians Pictorial Guide Vol 1 ISBN 978-0-473-15510-0

Introduction

The importance of the modern beauty therapist and aesthetician possessing basic cosmetic chemistry knowledge is becoming increasingly evident with modern body and skin care cosmetics rapidly encroaching upon the medical field with an ever-increasing range of truly effective products.

In addition to requiring accurate skin diagnosis skills, the therapist of the future will need to know with a degree of accuracy, what the effects of prescribed products and treatments will be when administered to specific skin conditions.

True cosmetic chemistry concerns itself not only with what is in our skin care and cosmetic products, but what chemical occurrences are happening in and around the various cells within the skin and how the chemicals in the cosmetics interact with the skins own chemistry.

In this book, we will examine the ingredients most commonly found in modern cosmetic products, and explain their actions and roles in the formulations. We will explain the relevant chemical events that occur in the cells and systems of the skin, and relate product composition to those events, and the effect they may have on specific conditions of the skin.

Cosmetic formulations are generally complex, however, for the purpose of this publication, we will try to simplify the structure of the compositions by only examining the aspects of data that is relevant to the beauty therapist/aesthetician.
Not all skin conditions can be addressed in this one book, so I will be concentrating on the skin conditions and related chemicals/active ingredients that influence them that we encounter in our clinics and practices most often. I have avoided controversial issues, myths and truths.

The information in this book has been sourced from scientific papers and cosmetic industry literature from America, Europe and Australasia, and is the most current information available at the time of writing. (August 2009), and I recognise that some more recent innovations since that time may have escaped my attention.

Florence Barrett-Hill
August 2009

Chapter one

Cosmetic Chemistry

- Making sense of the label
- Formulation basics
- Base ingredients
- Active ingredients
- Sun protection

Cosmetic Chemistry

Making sense of the label

A question I am often asked is "what is the difference between a product my client can buy in a supermarket or department store to what I sell in my clinic"? Do "clinic only" products have more therapeutic properties? Are department store products really able to perform the miracles they claim? If so, how? These are valid questions, and the purpose of this book is to help you navigate your way around cosmetic formulations so you can make a considered judgement without the influence of marketing hype.

When skin care product providers train clinicians in a chosen product range, a lot of time is spent discussing actives and actions, benefits and positives for both clinic treatments and retail products. Then time may be spent on what the competitor's products may or may not contain, but very little time if any is spent on the formula in general and the chemicals through which the actives are dispersed. Sometimes we are so concerned with the properties of the active ingredients that we disregard what else is in the formula. It is not uncommon for the "vehicle" or medium of a cream or formulation to be the part we should be concerned about with regard to some skin conditions. Those of you familiar with the philosophy of the Pastiche Method® will know the secret is to relate as much as you can to skin structure and function, using your knowledge of skin and of course, cosmetic chemistry when replying to questions from your clients.

Analysing a label

One of the most valuable skills of a skin care professional is the ability to "read" or understand a formulation. This allows us to determine a number of things including the quality of the product and it's intended purpose. Understanding the label allows us to determine if the formulation is contributing to a skin condition we may be attempting to diagnose, or if a particular product is appropriate for use under certain conditions. We can only do this if we know what is in the product, what those components do, and their respective properties. Thankfully in most countries, all cosmetic companies are required to list the ingredients on their products.

There may be some variation on these regulations, but those of the EU, USA, Japan, Canada, Australia and New Zealand follow this regulation.

The ingredients will be listed by the approved names found in the International Nomenclature of Cosmetic Ingredients (INCI). published by the Personal Care Products Council.

Cosmetic labels such as the example on the next page show ingredients listed in order of quantity in the overall formula, the first being the predominant ingredient the last being the least. This formula (and most others) will contain various classes of ingredients including:

- Solvents
- Conditioning ingredients
- Adjusting agents (texture & body)
- Fragrance

- Surfactants
- Preservatives
- Active ingredients
- Colour

Colour & Fragrance
Preservatives/antioxidants
Active ingredients
Processing aids
Base emulsion

There are many ingredients in formulations that perform specific functions that can be classified in to groups. The quantity of each group varies with the type of formulation.

Understanding formulations by reading the label

A practical component of this book will be to follow our example formulation below. It is a commonly used over the counter (OTC) cosmetic that is labelled and marketed as an anti-ageing product.
This cream is sold in supermarkets, department and drug stores (pharmacies) around the world and many of your clients may have used it.
What we are going to do is follow this formulation throughout the first chapter, learning about each part of the formulation and at the end of each segment, summarise what you have read and relate that new knowledge to this formulation. We will be asking questions and identifying any shortcomings or good points you may discover. If you do not already own a dictionary of cosmetic ingredients, I recommend one of the two listed below in the "recommended reading" sidebar.

> Ingredients: Aqua, Glycerine, Niacinamide, Cetyl alcohol, Propylene glycol, Petrolatum, Cyclopentasiloxane, Isopropyl palmitate, Panthenol, Tocopherol acetate, Tocopherol, Camellia sinensis, Ceramide 3, Stearyl alcohol, Myristyl alcohol, Propylene glycol stearate, Titanium dioxide, Palmitic acid, Stearic acid, Dimethicone, Carbomer, Steareth-21, Steareth-2, Disodium EDTA, Sodium hydroxide, Aluminim hydroxide, Phenoxyethanol, Imidazolidinyl urea, Methylparaben, Propylparaben, Benzyl alcohol, Parfum, Hexyl cinnamal, Linalool, Hydroxyisohexyl 3-cyclohexene carboxaldehyde, Butylphenol methylpropional, Alpha-isomethyl ionone, Hydroxycitronellal, Geraniol, Citronellol, Limonene.

Whenever you see the symbol above, we will be reviewing our sample formulation and discussing the ingredients just presented in the text.

Reading a label

Before we get in to the detail of various classes of ingredients, we need to understand the basics of reading a cosmetic label. Specifically how to decipher all of the information, to put it in bite size pieces for analysis. The following process usually works well:

1. Begin by listing the ingredients as they are written numbering them through from first to last.
2. The next step is to determine what class the various ingredients fall into. This will help you understand the formula better, and in time you will learn what all these ingredients do.
   Note: Begin at the bottom of the list. These will usually be colours, fragrance and preservatives. You can see in our example label above (and over the page) that these ingredients can take up as many as three lines on the list. (But will still be the least as a percentage of the total)
3. Next, try to identify the active ingredients. If you can't at this stage, move to the next step and return after step 5.
4. Now look at what you have got left: go to the top of the label and begin with the first, which is often water. What comes next is going to be the next highest quantity ingredient and so on.
5. The balance of the formulation is what the actives are dispersed through, and by working your way through the balance of ingredients, you will generally be able to determine the overall quality, purpose, price window and from a cosmetic "timeline", whether it is modern, traditional or outdated.

Important note:

Where the active ingredients are positioned in the list will give you some indication of the percentage in the formula, but keep in mind that some actives can often only be used in small quantities to retain their positive effect and not become toxic or oxidising. Just because there is a small quantity does not mean they will have less effect.
Products that follow standard USA labelling rules show anything above 1% concentration in the formula listed in order, and many ingredients below 1% can have a significant impact. Ingredients above 3%, however will usually provide the bulk of the aesthetic and performance characteristics.

Recommended reading:

A Consumer's Dictionary of Cosmetic Ingredients (Ruth Winter)
ISBN 978-1-4000-5233-2

Milady's Skin Care and Cosmetics Ingredients Dictionary (Third edition)
ISBN 978-1-4354-8020-9

Advanced Professional Skin Care, Medical Edition
ISBN 978-0-9630-2113-7

Example formulation: a closer look

Below is the break down of the 42 ingredients in the formula from the previous page in order of volume in the mix. You can see from the breakdown, the list is quite substantial.
Of the 42 ingredients, almost 43% are fragrance and preservatives. The balance perform the functions of either holding the other ingredients together or forming the vehicle for the few active ingredients. As discussed, this is the list of ingredients that we will re-visit at various steps throughout the first chapter to assist you in understanding the how's, what's and why's of cosmetic formulations.
Use this chart as a quick reference guide to confirm actions of ingredients in the formulation.

Ingredient	Purpose/property	Ingredient	Purpose/property
1. Aqua	Water (solvent and carrier)	22. Steareth-21	Solubilising agent/surfactant
2. Glycerine	Humectant (Hygroscopic)	23. Steareth-2	Emulsifier/surfactant
3. Niacinamide	Vitamin B3 (niacin or nicotinic acid)	24. Disodium EDTA	Chelating agent (Binds metal ions)
4. Cetyl alcohol	Emollient, emulsifier, thickening agent	25. Sodium hydroxide	Reagent
5. Propylene glycol	Humectant (Hygroscopic)	26. Aluminim hydroxide	Opacifier (Colour additive)
6. Petrolatum	Occlusion (Hydrophobic)	27. Phenoxyethanol	Preservative
7. Cyclopentasiloxane	Emollient (Silicone)	28. Imidazolidinyl urea	Preservative
8. Isopropyl palmitate	Emollient, thickening agent	29. Methylparaben	Paraben preservative
9. Panthenol	Humectant, emollient (Pro-vitamin B5)	30. Propylparaben	Paraben preservative
10. Tocopherol acetate	Vitamin E acetate (Antioxidant)	31. Benzyl alcohol	Fragrance fixative, solvent, preservative
11. Tocopherol	Vitamin E (Antioxidant)	32. Parfum	Fragrance
12. Camellia sinensis	Polyphenolic Antioxidant	33. Hexyl cinnamal	Fragrance
13. Ceramide 3	Lipid (Bio-identical fatty acid)	34. Linalool	Fragrance
14. Stearyl alcohol	Emollient, emulsifier, thickener	36. Hydroxyisohexyl 3-cyclohexene carboxaldehyde (Lyral) Fragrance	
15. Myristyl alcohol	Emollient	37. Butylphenol methylpropional	Fragrance
16. Propylene glycol stearate	Surfactant, emollient, conditioner	38. Alpha – isomthyl Ionone	Fragrance
17. Titanium dioxide	Colouring, (white) sun protection	39. Hydroxycitronellal	Fragrance
18. Palmitic acid	Surfactant, emulsifier, emollient (FFA)	40. Geraniol	Fragrance
19. Stearic acid	Surfactant, emulsifier	41. Citronellol	Fragrance
20. Dimethicone	Emollient (Silicone)	42. Limonene	Fragrance
21. Carbomer	Emulsion stabilizer, thickening agent		

What makes a good formulation?

The intention of a good skin care formulation is to restore all natural skin barrier defence systems or to prevent further deterioration of the defence systems while improving skin health generally.
To re-create a "balanced skin" it is important to restore the density of the spinosum layer and support the health of the keratinocyte, as it is crucial in the formation of the epidermis and maintaining skin barrier defence systems. If a skin care formulation is compatible to skin structure and function, it will have a positive effect and be beneficial to the high number of cells and systems of the epidermis.
A well balanced formulation should have the following properties and benefits:

- Mimic skin structure & function and skin barrier defence systems
- Maintain skin barrier defence systems
- Be partially occlusive
- Possess antioxidant properties
- Vitamin replacing
- Supporting of enzyme activity
- Slow trans epidermal water loss (TEWL)
- Be saturating
- Possess restorative properties
- Repairing
- Have a balanced pH

> **"Cosmetically Pleasing"**
>
> This "smells and feels nice" specification must not be discounted. It has been one of the major measures of formula success for decades, even though the formula may have had minimal therapeutic effect.

Finding the active ingredients in the formula can be considered the easy part and is the most susceptible to interpretation and marketing hype; despite this, the active should positively mimic the cells and systems they are targeting. This property is known as being "biomimetic".
The balance of the formulation should also be compatible to cells and systems and many of the carriers, emollients and humectants could be considered actives in their own right if well chosen.

With the technology and knowledge of the skin's systems available to cosmetic formulators today, there should be no excuse for what could be considered poor formulations, however time and again, old fashioned and questionable formulations continue to be manufactured and marketed to the skin treatment industry. Of course, end user price will always be the driving force for a formulator, and the old proverb "you get what you pay for" is always true in this case.

Formulation basics

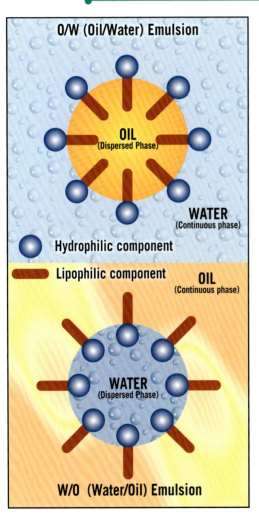

O/W (Oil/Water) Emulsion

OIL
(Dispersed Phase)

WATER
(Continuous phase)

Hydrophilic component

Lipophilic component

OIL
(Continuous phase)

WATER
(Dispersed Phase)

W/O (Water/Oil) Emulsion

Emulsions

These are one of the most common forms of cosmetic products. You find them in skin lotions, make-up, and even hair products. By definition, an emulsion is a dispersion of two or more immiscible (normally incapable of being mixed) materials, where one phase, known as the internal or dispersed phase, is dissolved in the continuous or external phase.

Simple cosmetic emulsions are classified as:

- Oil in water emulsion. (o/w) Low volume of oil in large volume of water.
- Water in oil emulsion. (w/o) Low volume of water in large volume of oil.
- Water in silicone (w/si emulsion) Example: a hand cream or barrier cream.
- Multiple emulsions such as oil in water in oil (w/o/w) are also possible.
- Oil free; these include solutions and gels. (Refer page 19 for details)

Oil in water emulsions are usually the most common in formulations due to lower production cost, ease of application and light texture. (Typical use: moisturiser)
In order to create an oil in water emulsion (with adequate stability), something must be done to overcome the interfacial tension between the two phases.
This can be achieved by simple mixing; however even mixing at very high rates is not enough to provide long term stability.
Simple mixed emulsions tend to revert to the stable state of oil separated from water, and so another ingredient called an ***emulsifier*** (or combination of emulsifiers) is needed to stabilise droplets of the dispersed phase.

What is an emulsifier?

Emulsifiers, or "surface active agents" are absorbed in the interface between the two liquids, forming a film between both substances: due to their structure, the polar part of the emulsifier molecule has an affinity with water and the non-polar part (fatty or oil chain) is attracted to the fatty phase.
The emulsifier forces one of the liquids into separate drops, suspended and dispersed within the other liquid. As these droplets are "guarded" by the emulsifier molecules surrounding them, they are kept apart from each other, ensuring the two substances do not separate but are kept in a stable mixture, enabling two usually non-mixable ingredients to mix together.

Surfactants and emulsifiers

Most emulsifiers can be considered surfactants or "surface-active agents". This property means that they are able to reduce the surface tension of water.

What makes an emulsifier "surface active" is related to the size of the hydrophilic (water-loving or polar) portion of a molecule, compared to the size of the lipophilic (oil-loving or non-polar) portion. The illustration below left is a typical emulsifying molecule.

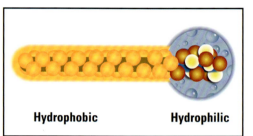

Hydrophobic   **Hydrophilic**

Surfactants in cosmetics can many functions:

- Emulsifiers: for creams and lotions
- Detergents: for cleansing
- Conditioning agents: in skin or hair care products
- Solubilisers: for perfumes and flavours
- Wetting agents: in perms

Surfactants are surface-active agents

Surfactants have a surface-active ion that is either positively or negatively charged, or contains no charge. The ionic charge is the key when classifying surfactants and emulsifiers, as the properties differ according to their ionic charge as well as the fatty acid that makes up the oil-soluble portion of the surface-active agent.

The toxic properties of the surfactants vary by type and it has been found that cationic surfactants tend to be more irritating than anionic surfactants and anionic surfactants more irritating than non-ionic surfactants.

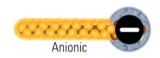

Anionic

Anionic surfactants

Anionic surfactants are negatively charged: these are the most commonly used cosmetic emulsifiers because they are cheap and stable. This is the most widely used type of surfactant for laundering, dishwashing liquids and shampoos because of its excellent cleaning properties and high foaming potential.

Common examples of anionic surfactants:

- Sodium lauryl sulphate
- Sodium dodecyl sulfate
- Ammonium lauryl sulfate, and other alkyl sulfate salts
- Sodium laureth sulfate, also known as sodium lauryl ether sulfate
- Alkyl benzene sulfonate

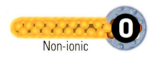

Non-ionic

Non-ionic surfactants

Non-ionic emulsifiers are often used in skin-care emulsions for their safety and low reactivity, and are uncharged: they do not dissociate into positive or negative ionic components when dissolved in water and can be used with either cationic or anionic emulsifiers as auxiliary emulsifiers.

They are also compatible with all other classes of surfactants and are soluble and effective in the presence of high concentrations of electrolytes, acids and alkalis.

Glycerine is a common example of a non-ionic surfactant, and is added to cosmetic emulsions for its hygroscopic humectant properties. It is the backbone of a class of emulsifiers called glyceryl esters and glyceryl monostearates.

Common non-ionic surfactants include:

- Alkyl poly (ethylene oxide)
- Copolymers of poly (ethylene oxide) and poly (propylene oxide) (commercially called Poloxamers or Poloxamines)
- Alkyl polyglucosides, including: Octyl glucoside, Decyl maltoside
- Fatty alcohols: Cetyl alcohol, Oleyl alcohol
- Cocamide MEA, Cocamide DEA, Polysorbates: Tween 20™ and Tween 80™.

Amphoteric surfactants

Amphoteric surfactants (also known as zwitterionic surfactants) contain dual functional groups in the same molecule, which, depending on pH, allows them to exist in anionic, non-ionic and cationic states. Amphoteric surfactants maintain their compatibility with all other types of surfactants over a wide pH range. Amphoterics are also known to be milder than traditional primary surfactants and are often incorporated in formulations specifically to mitigate the effects of harsher primary surfactants. The major applications for this class of surfactant are shampoos and body washes.

Typical examples include:

- Sodium cocoamphoacetate
- Sodium cocoamphopropionate,
- Disodium cocoamphodiacetate
- Disodium cocoamphodipropionate

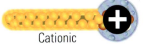
Cationic

Cationic surfactants

Cationic surfactants (ammonium compounds) are poorly tolerated by most skins and are now rarely used in quality skin care products. If you do see these types of surfactants in a product intended for the face, I would question the supplier and reconsider its application and use. However, they will still be seen in many household and laundry cleaning products.

Common cationic surfactants include:

- Ammonium lauryl sulfate. (Has high irritant potential)
- Dodecyl trimethylammonium bromide.
- Cetyl trimethylammonium bromide
- Cetylpyridinium chloride
- Polyethoxylated tallow amine
- Benzalkonium chloride
- Benzethonium chloride

PEGS (polyethylene glycol) as emulsifiers and surface active agents

These are synthetic plant glycols, polyethylene glycols, and polymers of ethylene oxide.
PEG is popular and versatile as it is soluble in water, methanol, benzene, and dichloromethane, but is considered by some as old fashioned. It is however, still widely used in all types of cosmetics and medications.
PEG compounds are used as binders, solvents, emollients, plasticisers, bases, carriers, emulsifiers and dispersants; it is because of this wide use that PEGS are an important part of any chemist's/ formulator's palette.

MPEGS

Methoxypolyethylene glycols are another range of water soluble polymers with similar properties to PEGS.
The numbering sequence for molecular weight and melting point is the same as PEGs.

The numbers that are often included in the names of PEGs indicate their average molecular weights and melting points. The range of PEGS in cosmetics is from 200 - 600 depending on the thickness of consistency required. An example is PEG 400: with molecular weight of 400 daltons.

The number also refers to the liquidity: the higher the number, the higher the melting point and the firmer the composition. PEG 400, for instance has a melting point of around 4-6° C, (39-46° F) so will be quite thin in consistency. PEG 600 with a melting point of 20-25° C (68-77° F) will be thicker while in the tube or pot, but become thinner when on the skin surface due to body heat.

Controversy about PEGS is that the low molecular polyethylene glycols from 200 to 400 may cause skins to be itchy and dry, however the higher weights are not known sensitisers.

PEGS with numbers below 200 generally refer to derivatives of/or blends with other ingredients, so there will be much less of the polyethylene glycol in the substance than the full number value.
An example is PEG-20 Dilurate, which is polyethylene glycol and lauric acid. The number associated with the name is the average number of units of ethylene oxide (PEG) that has been used in the chemical reaction with other substances to produce the material.

Biosurfactants

Also known as microbial surface active agents, these "green" complex organic surfactants are used as emulsifiers, foaming agents, solubilisers, wetting agents, cleansers, antimicrobial agents, and mediators of enzyme actions.

Biosurfactants are high molecular weight lipid complexes in the form of glycolipids, lipopeptides and phospholipids. What makes them so different from their synthetic counterparts is their origin, as they are created by fermentation processes, incorporating enzymes and bacteria. In other words, they are produced by micro-organisms.

Emulsifier free?

Emfulsifier free formulations that mimic skin structure and function are now being used for skin treatment therapy products.
See page 29 for more information

The major properties of biosurfactants are biodegradability, biocompatability, digestibility and generally low toxicity, which means they exhibit extremely low skin irritation. They are also very small, in the nanometer range. Bio-surfactants produced from yeast and vegetable oils have been shown to exhibit similar moisturising properties to natural ceramides, however they are more expensive because of the complex processes of manufacture.

Surfactin sodium salt is an example of a modern anionic lipopeptide biosurfactant, and Rhamnolipid is an example of a high-tech glycolipid.

Quality of emulsifier or surfactant will be reflected in the retail price

A basic understanding of emulsion systems will help determine how a product is put together, and usually indicates the intended market and price-point.

In the ideal world, an emulsifier should be sourced from natural ingredients such as vegetable oils and other vegetable-based raw materials.

Unfortunately, nature provides us with only a few emulsifiers such as lecithin and egg yolk and in the early days of cosmetics, these did not always perform consistently enough for commercial viability. Soybean lecithin and rice bran oil is still the benchmark today for skin compatibility. Other emulsifiers from the food industry are being successfully used for commercial cosmetics products, with examples sourced from coconut and palms oils.

An example of the price structure and differences in common emulsifiers are listed by their types and price per kilo (In 2009) in the chart opposite. You will see the obvious relationship between price, performance and quality.

Typical emulsifiers and their approximate cost as a raw material

Vegetal

Vegetal chemistry is, as the name suggests based on vegetable substances sourced as a raw material.
An example is glucose derived from corn and emollient sourced from coconut.
There is a price to pay for this, as the more rare and unsustainable the raw material, the more expensive.

Cetearyl glucoside €46.87 per kilo
A modern emulsifier made according to ecological principles with no chemicals or solvents used, it is ideal for making light creams, lotions & conditioners. The water-binding part of vegetal is sourced from glucose, which is extracted from corn and the fatty element of vegetal is sourced from coconut.

Sodium stearoyl lactylate €29.04 per kilo
Vegetable-based emulsifier for creams and lotions, derived from lactic acid and vegetable-based stearic acid. It produces a professional cosmetic product.

Glyceryl monostearate €26.52 per kilo
A vegetable-based emulsifier made from stearic and palmitic acid. A good substitute for vegetal in creams and lotions. Great for making light creams.

Cetyl alcohol €19.91 per kilo
Used as a stabiliser for other emulsifiers. Made from palm kernel oil fatty acid (Palmitic acid), which is treated with liquid gas so that the free oxygen (O) atom is removed. Cetyl alcohol makes creams and lotions firmer and gives them consistency.

Surfactants for cleansing

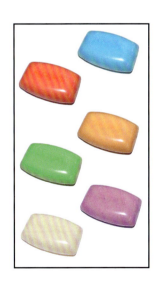

The words surfactant and foam are characteristics often considered as part of the cleansing process. Most cleansing is accomplished with a soap, which is obtained through the chemical reaction between a fat and an alkali, resulting in a fatty acid salt with detergent properties.
Modern refinements have attempted to adjust its alkaline pH, possibly resulting in less skin irritation and to incorporate substances that prevent the formation of calcium fatty acid salts in hard water, more commonly known as soap scum.
Even so, modern soap is still basically a blend of tallow and nut oil, or the fatty acids derived from these products, generally in a ratio of 4:1. Increasing this ratio results in "super-fatted" soaps designed to leave an oily film behind on the skin. (Traditional Dove® soap is a good example)
Additives to soap are also responsible for a characteristic appearance, feel and smell. Examples are:

- Lanolin and paraffin may be added to moisturising syndet soaps to create a super fatted soap.
- Sucrose and glycerine can be added to create a transparent bar, such as the "Pears" soap.
- The use of olive oil instead of tallow or nut oils distinguishes the classic "Castile" soap.
- Titanium dioxide is added in concentrations as high as 0.3% to opacify the bar and to increase its optical whiteness, and other pigments, such as aluminium lakes, can colour the bar without producing an undesirable coloured foam.
- The use of foam builders, such as sodium carboxy-methylcellulose and other cellulose derivatives, can make the soaps lather feel creamy.
- Perfume in concentrations of 2% or more also can be added to ensure that the soap bar retains a pleasant smell until completely used.

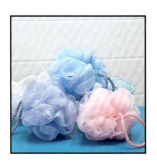

Bar and liquid cleansers

- True soaps composed of long chain fatty acid alkali salts with a pH of 9 -10.
- Combars composed of alkaline soaps to which surface active agents have been added, also with a pH of 9 -10.
- Syndet (synthetic detergent) bars composed of synthetic detergents and fillers that contain less than 10% soap and have an adjusted pH of 5.5 - 7.0.

Medicated soaps

These types may contain benzoyl peroxide, sulphur, or resorcinol antibacterials, such as triclocarban or triclosan. Triclocarban is excellent at eradicating gram-positive organisms, and triclosan eliminates both gram-positive and gram-negative bacteria. (Not always a good thing) These soaps generally exhibit a pH between 9 - 10 and may cause irritation if the skin is compromised. Moisturising syndet bar soaps contain sodium lauryl isethionate with a pH adjusted between 5 - 7 by lactic or citric acid. These products are less irritating to the skin and are sometimes labelled beauty bars.

Foaming facial & body washes

Foam is the delivery medium that is beginning to be preferred by consumers as it is associated with a more effective cleansing result and adds a touch of luxury. Body washes are replacing soap for use in the daily shower, and these are marketed using all of the tricks and perceived benefits of colour and smell, with "natural" ingredients leading the way.

These foams are applied with a shower washing "net" to break apart the emulsion through the incorporation of generous amounts of air and water. These nets do not support bacterial growth and are easily sanitised.

High amounts of petroleum can be incorporated in body wash emulsions to improve skin dryness and hydration, and it should be remembered that the quality of them varies considerably.

Commonly used detergents in bar-type soap	Detergents in liquid/gel cleansers
• Sodium cocoate	• Sodium laureth sulfate
• Sodium tallowate	• Cocoamido propyl betaine
• Sodium palm kernelate	• Lauramide DEA
• Sodium stearate	• Sodium cocoyl isethionate
• Sodium palmitate	• Disodium laureth sulfosuccinate
• Triethanolamine stearate	
• Sodium cocoyl isethionate	
• Sodium isethionate	
• Sodium dodecyl benzene sulfonate	
• Sodium cocoglyceryl ether sulfonate	

Surfactants sourced from vegetable lipo-peptide salts

Coconut and soy protein are commonly being used as surfactants, and are appearing in facial cleansing and hair products.

- Potassium salt of lauroyl hydrolysed wheat protein
- Sodium & sodium TEA salts of cocoyl hydrolysed soya protein
- Potassium salt of cocoyl hydrolysed rice protein

pH of cosmetic products

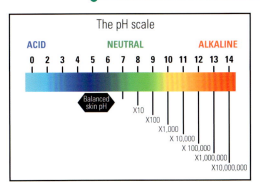

The pH scale

ACID **NEUTRAL** **ALKALINE**

0 2 3 4 5 6 7 8 9 10 11 12 13 14

Balanced
skin pH

X10
X100
X1,000
X 10,000
X 100,000
X1,000,000
X10,000,000

pH is a logarithmic scale. A difference of one pH unit is
equivalent to a ten-fold difference in hydrogen ion concentration

pH explained

The term pH stands for potential hydrogen and refers to the degree of acidity or
alkalinity of a substance. This is measured by the amount of free hydrogen atoms
and expressed by the pH.

The pH scale is a measurable reference point of how acidic or alkaline a
substance is, with it's scale ranging from 0 to 14.

A pH of 7 is neutral, with a pH less than 7 considered acidic, and a pH greater
than 7 considered alkaline.

The pH scale is logarithmic and this means that each whole pH value in ten times
more acidic or alkaline than the next higher or lower value.

For example, pH 4 is ten times more acidic than pH 5 and 100 times (10 times 10)
more acidic than pH 6. The same applies for pH values above 7, each of which is
ten times more alkaline than the next lower whole value. For example, pH 10 is
ten times more alkaline than pH 9 and 100 times (10 times 10) more alkaline than pH 8.

Skin pH and the acid mantle

There are many skin conditions we see every day in our clinics where the practices of our clients
have unwittingly been contributing to the development or acceleration of their conditions by using
inappropriate cleansers (excessive pH) and practices and when we are conducting our initial
consultations, the importance of the client bringing their cleansers with them cannot be understated.
A major contributing cause of their condition could well be in their daily use products.
Washing skin with high alkalinity soaps or cleansers can cause the temporary loss of acid mantle, and
repetitive washing will change the skin pH, affecting the stratum corneum and barrier functions.

In the early 90's it was very fashionable to test the pH of clients skin's, and it was included in my
Advanced Skin Analysis training as part of the consultation at that time. Over the years I have found
that the variables in skin pH over the course of a 24 hour period were enough to show that the pH of
a skin was not consistent enough, and to try to use the pH as a skin diagnostic tool was a waste of
time.

A healthy skin with an intact acid mantle has a superb buffering capacity and adjusts quickly,
restoring the acid pH of the surface. If however, the skin is not healthy and the client is cleansing
twice a day with products that contain high foaming, low quality surfactants, the skin will find it
very difficult to rebalance the pH, and over time will become aggressed and the skin barrier defence
systems break down. (A compromised skin)

pH Testing of a product

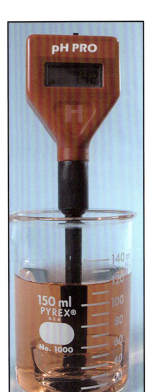

Testing of the client's product during the consultation process proved to be very successful and often
I was able to pin point a particular bath soap or cleansing gel as being too alkaline to be used on a
twice-daily basis, which is what is too often done.
Testing a product with litmus paper is not professional enough for a clinic and it would be better to
use more scientific (and credible) electronic methods of reading pH.
Thankfully these products are affordable and for a small investment you have raised the credibility
profile of your clinic considerably.
It is best to test soaps cleansers and toners first then if you feel it is required, also test day and night
creams.

The reason for this is due to the mess that creams can make of the pH-testing electrode. It is best to leave the testing of those substances that require careful cleansing of the probe until last.

I have found that almost all "beauty therapy" products have a balanced pH and will generally present no surprises. Instead, make yourself more familiar with the domestic retail products and be more vigilant when testing them.

pH Balanced: What does it mean?

On the packaging of shampoos, lotions and creams the term "pH balanced" so often appears. The phrase "pH balanced" means very little because it doesn't really tell you about what's in the formulation, they are "marketing words" that your customer sees on TV and reads in magazines. For a product to have a consistent pH very often chemical buffers have been used to maintain the chosen pH. This means that it won't matter what else is put into the formulation as the pH will stay constant. Please do not think this is necessarily a bad thing; rather consider it as part of the formulation's stability.

The following chemicals are commonly used as buffers in cosmetic formulations:

- Aminomethyl propanol
- Phosphoric acid
- Sodium citrate
- Tetrahydroxypropyl ethylenediamine
- Triethanolamine

- Citric acid
- Potassium phosphate
- Sodium hydroxide
- Potassium hydroxide
- Dipotassium phosphate

To illustrate the spectrum of pH in everyday products, the table below shows the test results of a selection of products brought to one of my cosmetic chemistry seminars.

pH	Product	Type
6.7	Natures Organics	Foaming face wash
6.8	Palmolive Softwash	Liquid soap
6.9	Dove beauty bar	Bar soap
7.2	Bubble Magic	Bubble bath
8.0	Environ B active Sebuwash	Facewash
8.0	Redwin Sorbolene	Bar soap
8.0	Gatineau Nutriactive	Cleanser
8.2	Clean & Clear	Facial wash
9.5	Palmolive Aroma Crème	Bar soap
9.6	Palmolive Naturals	Bar soap
9.6	Radox herbal bath	Bath salts
9.7	J&J baby soap	Bar soap
9.9	Honey kids soap	Children's soap
10.0	Nelum Sandalwood	Bar soap
10.0	Lux supreme cream	Bar soap
10.3	Simple soap	Bar soap
10.3	Sunlight pure soap	Bar soap
10.5	Nivea Crème bar	Bar soap

Formulation review

Our review product is a well-known cream, marketed and labelled as an anti-wrinkle, firming night cream that offers the benefits of smoothing fine lines and wrinkles. This is the first of seven reviews we will undertake to ascertain whether the ingredients listed are actually capable of delivering these claims, and assess the suitability for specific skin conditions/types.

To make the learning process easier, the ingredients under discussion in each review will be highlighted in red (As in the in our list below). After each review, the ingredients previously discussed will become faded or grey. This will avoid confusion by helping identify ingredients not yet reviewed, which will remain listed in strong black text.

The highlighted ingredients in this review are surfactants and pH buffers, and now that you have read this section about those particular substances, the questions should be easier for you to answer.

1. Are the surfactants highlighted of high or low quality? (Remember that the quality of the surfactant is usually reflected by the retail price)

2. Can you identify the ionic group of the surfactants used? (ie: cationic, non-ionic, amphoteric, etc.)

3. Would these surfactants benefit a mature ageing skin?

4. Can you identify the pH regulators?

Ingredients: Aqua, Glycerine, Niacinamide, Cetyl alcohol, Propylene glycol, Petrolatum, Cyclopentasiloxane, Isopropyl palmitate, Panthenol, Tocopherol acetate, Tocopherol, Camellia sinensis, Ceramide 3, Stearyl alcohol, Myristyl alcohol, Propylene glycol stearate, Titanium dioxide, Palmitic acid, Stearic acid, Dimethicone, Carbomer, Steareth-21, Steareth-2, Disodium EDTA, Sodium hydroxide, Aluminim hydroxide, Phenoxyethanol, Imidazolidinyl urea, Methylparaben, Propylparaben, Benzyl alcohol, Parfum, Hexyl cinnamal, Linalool, Hydroxyisohexyl 3-cyclohexene carboxaldehyde, Butylphenol methylpropional, Alpha-isomethyl ionone, Hydroxycitronellal, Geraniol, Citronellol, Limonene.

This check list will help you compare our review ingredients to the desirable criteria of a well balanced formulation, and ingredient type specifications.
Use the check list to confirm your assessment of what you have learned so far.

Did you draw the same conclusions?

Compatability check list

	Surfactant	Emulsifier	pH buffer	Anionic	Non-ionic	Amphoteric	Biomimetic	Occlusive	Antioxidant	Vitamin replacing	Restorative	Hydrating	Repair	Compromised skin
Cetyl alcohol		✓			✓									
Stearyl alcohol	✓				✓									
Stearic acid	✓			✓										✓
Steareth-2		✓			✓									✓
Steareth-21	✓				✓									

Ingredient specifications   Desirable criteria

Humectants-saturation-hydration

An examination of the water content of various epidermal layers show that the water content of the basal layer is around 70%, with significantly less (Around 13% at the stratum corneum) in the outermost layers. The quantity at these outer layers will depend to some extent on the relevant ambient humidity, the lipid phases of the bilayers, an intact acid mantle, and a healthy strong corneocyte.

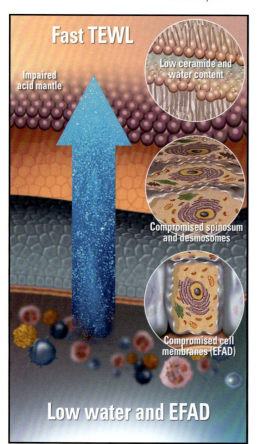

Fast TEWL

Impaired acid mantle

Low ceramide and water content

Compromised spinosum and desmosomes

Compromised cell membranes (EFAD)

Low water and EFAD

Diffusion of water through the skin (TEWL)

Trans-epidermal water loss (TEWL) is a term that is generally non-specific, but it is the mainstay of studying factors that affect the moisture of the skin.
For those who understand the physics; TEWL = delta RH/100x D x AF x 1/A.
Delta RH is the difference between the incoming and effluent relative humidity.
D is the weight of water per litre of saturated steam at the temperature of the air passing over the skin in milligrams. AF is the volumetric airflow rate in 1 hour.
A is the area of skin in centimetres squared.

Oil and water work in synergy

Oil and water work in synergy and the hydrophilic phase of an oil molecule will always require water to remain lipophilic.
To retain water in the lower layers of the epidermis and the stratum corneum, the oil phases of the epidermis must be intact. These oil phases are part of the skin barrier defence systems, with the acid mantle the first, the hydrophobic keratin cells of the stratum corneum the second, and the bilayers the third.

Any disruption of these three skin barrier defence systems will lead to an increase in TEWL (evaporation of water) this, in turn, will cause in impaired enzyme activity resulting in abnormal desquamation, poor alignment of bilayers, lipid dryness, and an impaired acid mantle, as well as hot, burning, and itchy skin.

Oil sits on top of water

Lack of "free water": (impaired enzyme activity, AKA "dehydration")
A lack of free water within the epidermis has for decades been described by the cosmetic industry as "dehydration", with a majority of creams sold for this condition being o/w based creams with the water phase being targeted as the moisturising (water replacement) phase.
The most frequently used chemicals for this purpose have the ability to attract water, (from both the air and lower levels of the epidermis) and include chemicals in the hydroxyl groups (-OH) such as glycerine, sorbitol and butylene or other glycols.

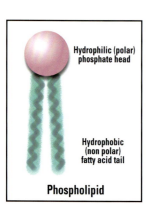

Hydrophilic (polar) phosphate head

Hydrophobic (non polar) fatty acid tail

Phospholipid

Prior to the 1990's, very little emphasis was placed on the oil phase (emollient phase) of day-use moisturising creams, which would actually play a significant role in temporarily replacing the lipid phases and help slow TEWL (evaporation). This disregard for the oil phase often resulted in the chosen emollient being of poor quality and only chosen for its "slip" and occlusive properties. (Unfortunately, there are still products on the market with this criteria)
It was not until the early 90's, when ceramides were first used in formulations appeared that there was a change of mindset by the cosmetic industry. The step was revolutionary in that, by realising

that if the natural oil phases of the skin (epidermic lipids) were improved, TEWL (evaporation) would be slowed resulting in a higher percentage of free water remaining in the lower more active layers of the epidermis. By simply using an active that would more closely mimic skin lipid physiology, (ceramides) the hydration of the skin was increased and lasted around 36% longer than any other conventional creams on the market at the time.

Most day moisturisers are still oil in water (o/w) based creams, however the more current, better formulated ones feature an emollient phase of higher quality and greater affinity to epidermic lipids. The humectant phase is generally based on amino acids or other bio-mimicking water solubles (NMF) of the epidermis, to provide a superior saturating and hydrating effect.

Stratum corneum water-soluble (SCWS)

Stratum corneum water-solubles (SCWS)	
Free amino acids	40.0%
Pyrrolidone carboxylic acid (PCA)	2.0%
Urea	7.0%
NH3, uric acid, glucosamine & creatinine	1.5%
Sodium	5.0%
Calcium	1.5%
Potassium	4.0%
Magnesium	1.5%
Phosphate	0.5%
Chloride	6.0%
Lactate	12.0%
Citrate, formate	0.5%
Unidentified	8.0%

Many of the modern, "effective" moisturising formulations use substances that are closely related or mimic the water solubles (NMF/extracellular fluid) of the stratum corneum. The composition of these water solubles comprise of approx 40% amino acids and 30% cellular waste, with a further 25% being the essential elements to the function of the epidermis. (See sidebar at left)

It is some of these essentials that are being used in cosmetic formulations as humectants or film formers with saturating and hydrating abilities. (More detail in chapter 2)

Pyrrolidone carboxylic acid (PCA) and sodium PCA (na PCA)

Sodium PCA is hygroscopic, attracting moisture from the air. It is highly water-absorbent, holding several times its weight in water, which makes it an excellent humectant. It is a stronger hydrating agent with saturation abilities than the traditional compounds used for this purpose, such as glycerine, propylene glycol, or sorbitol.

Calcium

This essential element regulates cell turnover of the keratinocyte, regulates lipid (lamellar) formation and continual efficient barrier functions. Clients with very lipid dry skins and essential fatty acid deficiency (EFAD) respond well to topically applied calcium treatment resulting in reduced cellular inflammation. Other calcium derivatives include calcium bentonite, calcium alginate, and calcium glucarate

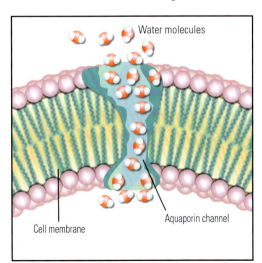

Aquaporin 3 is a direct pathway of ensuring water molecules gain intracellular access.

Magnesium & phosphate

Magnesium ions are essential for the function of the cells of all known living organisms, and are present in over 300 biochemical reactions in the human body. Consequently, its efficacy as a skin care ingredient is exciting, as it is easily assimilated by the lower epidermal layers, assisting in regeneration and healing of damaged skin cells. It is also a natural anti-allergen that supports healthy skin against cellular inflammation similar to calcium.

The different molecules that can be attached to magnesium seem to be endless, formulators understand that by having ion receptors for molecules such as magnesium, make it easier to "trick" or promote the cell to increase absorption of other substances. (An example is magnesium ascorbyl phosphate: vitamin C) The cell has many proteins throughout the membrane that selectively allow individual substances to pass through them. For magnesium or calcium they are specific ion receptors that act in the same way as aquaporin channels do for water. (Shown at left)

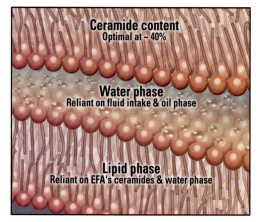

Ceramide content
Optimal at ~ 40%

Water phase
Reliant on fluid intake & oil phase

Lipid phase
Reliant on EFA's ceramides & water phase

Prevention of loss or replacement of epidermal water phases

It has been established that water is crucial to enzyme activity of the epidermis, to prevent crystallisation of the stratum corneum bilayer lipids, and for the alignment of the keratinocyte cell membrane phospholipid content.
A moisturiser should prevent or slow evaporation (slow TEWL) of water through the epidermis or it could replace water to the stratum corneum. This can be achieved by the use of chemicals that have humectant/saturation ability or be a non-polar lipid such as a phospholipid, a ceramide or an essential fatty acid. (EFA)

Saturation chemicals are film-forming

Saturation of the skin surface can be achieved by imparting a temporary barrier to the stratum corneum. Saturating chemicals are moisturisers/humectants of the new millennium; and these include agents that mimic skin structure and function, and include vitamins and botanicals.
Other ingredients commonly found are sodium hyaluronate (hyaluronic acid), pyrrolidone carboxylic acid (PCA), and ceramides; all are saturating and hydrating, (moisture givers) and leave more behind than they take.

Amino acids: the body's own saturating humectants

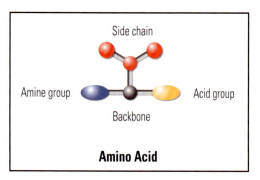

Side chain

Amine group

Acid group

Backbone

Amino Acid

The human body is composed mostly of water, with the second most common constituent being protein, or more specifically, "amino acid chains".
As mentioned, 40% of the water phase of the epidermis (SCWS/NMF) comprise of amino acids. For humans, there are nine essential amino acids and eleven non-essential amino acids.
From these twenty amino acids being combined & arranged into varying specific chains, the human body fabricates all proteins.
These are the basic building blocks that combine into literally thousands of complex protein, amino acid chains. Below are the twenty free amino acids of the epidermis that function as chemical messengers and as intermediates in metabolism.

Amino acids used by cosmetic formulators

- Alanine
- Arginine
- Asparagine
- Aspartic acid
- Cysteine
- Glutamic acid
- Glutamine
- Glycine
- Histidine
- Isoleucine
- Leucine
- Lysine
- Methionine
- Phenylalanine
- Proline
- Serine
- Threonine
- Tryptophan
- Tyrosine
- Valine

In cosmetic chemistry today, the "amino acid" has everyone's attention; it is from these chemicals that the advancement into anti-ageing cosmetics has come and the creation of actives such as "Matrixyl®" has evolved, from the manipulation of amino acids by combining them with fatty acids, such as palmitic acid.
The amino acids chosen come from a wide source of plant and synthetic ingredients, and extracting an amino acid component and understanding the role that it plays, or action that it may have on skin is relatively easy with today's science. See page 35 for more on amino acids and peptides.

Humectants

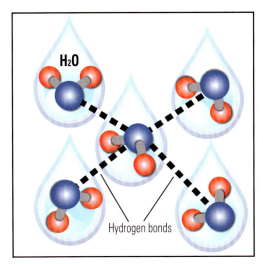

Hygroscopic action draws water molecules together

A humectant is any substance that is hygroscopic (ability to form hydrogen bonds with molecules of water) and can absorb water from both the air and from the lower layer of the epidermis. The transport of water to the upper stratum corneum (SC) temporarily increases the surface water level of skin (hydration). However, if the relevant ambient humidity is low, this water will be quickly evaporated into the atmosphere, leaving the stratum corneum without the free water it requires to function.

Humectants can make skin dryer and more aggressed

Humectants are usually molecules with one or more hydrophilic groups attached to them. These hydrophilic groups can either be:
- Aamines ($-NH3$) such as urea or amino acids.
- Carboxyl groups ($-COOH$) such as fatty acids or alpha hydroxy acids.
- Hydroxyl groups ($-OH$) such as glycerine, sorbitol and butylene or other glycols.

These lower molecular weighted glycols were thought at one time to approach the ideal in humectants, however because they do not perform well in low humidity conditions, they often contribute to a dry feeling.

If skin surface lipids are low, the use of humectants can further increase transepidermal water loss due to the hygroscopic properties mentioned. In addition, if the client is also suffering from internal dehydration and EFAD, the amount of fluid to draw on will be less, resulting in a severely irritated and aggressed skin surface. We can conclude that formulations containing large quantities of glycerine based humectants will have limited effect in a hot, dry environment on a compromised skin.

Choosing a cream

Understanding the weight of cream required for a particular task is key to ensuring your client is getting the best cream for the job.

During the consultation it would have been ascertained what the climates of work/play/at home environment are, and if the work environment has an artificial climate, (air conditioning) then the percentage of water in the air will usually be low and fast TEWL will occur if the skin is lipid dry or without a functioning acid mantle.

Therefore, the cream chosen for the day should impart a barrier to slow TEWL, maintaining hydration within the skin layers.

Conversely, if the "at home" environment has a humidity factor of over 65%, the reverse should apply, and a lighter weighted cream/gel would be recommended. Gels are a better option for outdoor, high humidity situations and will not over-hydrate the epidermis.

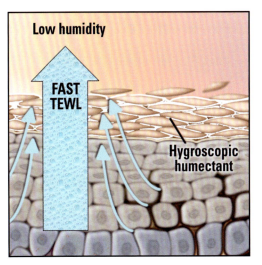

Low humidity

FAST TEWL

Hygroscopic humectant

Propylene glycols

The types used in cosmetics are usually a pharmaceutical grade of monopropylene glycol (PG or MPG) with a specified purity greater than 99.8%.
Although of high purity, they can still provoke skin irritation and sensitisation in products with as low as 2% concentration when skin is compromised.

Common humectants that absorb water from the air (hygroscopic)

- Butylene glycol
- Ethylene glycol
- Urea
- Diethylene glycol

- Glycerine
- Sorbitol trioleate
- Glycereth-26
- Methyl gluceth-20

- Propylene glycol
- Sorbic acid
- PEG-4 Octanoate

Humectants and compounds with film forming (Saturation & hydration giving) properties

- Tocopheryl linoleate
- Ceramides
- Hydroxypropyl chitosan
- Sphingolipids
- Carbamide
- Lactic acid
- Hydrolysed whole wheat protein
- Vegetable lipo-amino acid
- Soluble hydrolysed collagen/elastin

- ß glucan
- Sodium lactate
- Silk amino acids
- Phytalluronate
- Carbitol
- Sodium hyaluronate/hyaluronic acid
- Glycopolypeptides
- Colloidal oatmeal

- Sorbitol
- Hydrolysed wheat protein
- Phospholipids
- Corn oil unsaponifiable
- Polyglycerylmethacrylate
- Wheat amino acids
- Corn seed extract / fraction

Many of these compounds have hydrating and saturating abilities, with some retaining up to four hundred times their weight in water, and enabling excellent saturation of the water phase of the bilayers.

Wheat proteins help to reduce the irritating effect of surfactants and can still have foam-building and emulsifying actions superior to ingredients of animal origin.

Surface humectant and emollient abilities along with the unique amino acid profile make many of these wheat and oat derivatives a great contribution to the industry. (See more in the secretions section in chapter four.)

Marine based humectants

Algae and marine based actives have high amino acid contents that are beneficial for skin, with many of the algae's and sea water derivatives available to the beauty industry. Dead Sea and Moor Mud also have enormous therapeutic and absorbing properties, and these abilities mean that algae often have a greater medicinal spa application than beauty therapy.

Spirulina as a humectant

Spirulina is a microscopic blue-green algae. It is classified as a vegetable plankton with cells that form the shape of a coiled spring, thus the name spirulina, which means "little spiral".

Unlike other plants and animals, spirulina does not have complicated bodies and biochemistries to maintain, with it's total function is to produce protein, carbohydrates, vitamins, amino acids, and protective pigments.

Spirulina is high in amino acid content (all 9 essential amino acids) and essential fatty acids, including the much needed Omega 3 and 6 fatty acids.

Spirulina has taken the beauty industry by storm, with its high amino acids profile, essential fatty acids omega 3 & 6,14 minerals, over 2000 active enzymes, ßeta-carotene, B12, B1, B5 and B6, just to name a few.

The polyunsaturated oils in spirulina contain 21-29% GLA, making it one of nature's richest whole-food source of gamma linolenic acid.

Algae as a humectant

Each variety of seaweed possesses its own individual cocktail of elements, and cosmetic formulators are careful to choose the appropriate seaweed for the required function.

Regardless of whether algae are macerated or micronised, the benefits of algae in cosmetics are endless. All the sea's mineral substances are concentrated in seaweed cells, in a manner similar to a tiny chemical manufacturing plant. Algae are also a source of proteins, vitamins and antioxidants, as well as 9 amino acids, providing a synergy with the water solubles of the epidermis.

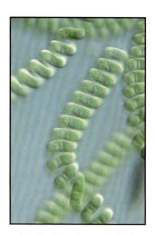

Spirulina is a microscopic fresh water algae that is one of nature's richest whole-food source of gamma linolenic acid.

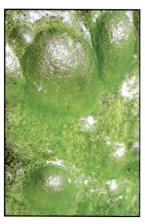

There are 9 amino acids found in algae, which is also a source of proteins, vitamins and antioxidants.

Xylose as a humectant

Xylose (or wood sugar) is becoming a popular humectant with department store brand products, with xylose derivatives and compounds commanding the most attention. (Example: Pro-Xylane®)
Also known by the names D-xylose and Xylose-L, the use of these monosaccarides is primarily as a water-binding agent, however it is when it is further refined, blended (with amino acids, vitamins and esters of natural fatty acids) and encapsulated (in liposomes) it attains more anti-ageing properties.
In this form, the resulting oligosaccharide containing xylose compounds are claimed to work by stimulating the synthesis of proteoglycans / glycosaminoglycans, with an improvement of all epidermal sub-systems as a consequence.

Oil-free emulsions

The definition of "oil-free" is not as simple as it first seems, as there are compounds that, while technically are oil-free by name, (the word oil does not appear in the name) still contain substances that exhibit oily properties. For the purposes of this discussion, we will only refer to substances that are considered strictly "oil free".

Oil free substances are usually solutions and gels that have a drying effect owing to the evaporation of solvent. Alcohol solutions are very drying because ethanol and other low molecular weight alcohols are volatile and evaporate rapidly. Whereas water solutions are only mildly drying because of the slower evaporation of water.
Gels are clear, non-oily solid products that consist of long chain molecules such as cellulose derivatives or carbomers along with a small amount of solvent (water, alcohol or acetone).
They are usually mildly drying owing to the evaporation of the solvent and are most useful for oily skin.

Note: An exception to the oil-free rule is essential oils. These are emollient esters, and do not behave like other oils and so can be properly included as an "oil free" product.

Oil-free or not oil-free?: The oil migration test

Not all "oil-free" moisturisers for cosmetics are oil free; some contain oil-like synthetics that can provoke acne-prone skin. So when you are not sure, how do you tell?
The trick is to dab a small sample of the mystery moisturiser on a piece of good-quality stationery (imprinted 25% cotton fibre). Leave it for approx. twenty-four hours, and then hold the paper up to daylight and check for oil rings. The extent of migration will correspond to the percent of oil in the cosmetic.

The properties of emulsion bases

The table below illustrates the properties of various emulsion bases. The extremes of types are from ointment types that sit on the surface and raise hydration levels by slowing evaporation of epidermal extracullular fluid (NMF) by occlusion, to quickly evaporating non-occlusive hygroscopic gels and water based solutions.

Moisturising		Neutral		Drying
Ointment bases Water free products	Water in oil emulsions w/o Oil based products	Oil in water emulsions o/w Water based products	Oil-free emulsions with emollient esters Glycerine & glycol bases	Strictly oil-free emulsions Gels and water solutions	Alcohol solutions Other volatile solutions

---

Carbomers

A series of polymers primarily made from acrylic acid. They are able to absorb and retain water, and can swell to many times their original volume. They are used to suspend or distribute an insoluble solid in a liquid, or help keep emulsions from separating into their oil/water phases.

Formulation review

Listed in our example formulation (highlighted in red) are the humectants that make up the water phase of the example cream. (You will note the previously discussed ingredients are now faded out)

As we have previously discussed, the price of a skin care product will usually be reflected by the quality of the surfactant, and the same holds true for the quality of the humectant. A better quality humectant will have more of an affinity with the water-soluble phase of the epidermis and epidermic skin lipids.

The amino acids, glucosamine and hyaluronic acids are examples of water soluble humectants compatible with the extracellular fluid (NMF) or the ground substance of the dermis.

1. Are any of the ingredient listed "skin compatible"?

2. Can you determine if the type of humectant is a " giver" type film former that leaves a water type substance in the skin layers, or is it a "taker" that draws water to the skins surface and from the atmosphere and ultimately evaporates quickly?

3. Are the humectants of high quality?

Ingredients: Aqua, Glycerine, Niacinamide, Cetyl alcohol, Propylene glycol, Petrolatum, Cyclopentasiloxane, Isopropyl palmitate, Panthenol, Tocopherol acetate, Tocopherol, Camellia sinensis, Ceramide 3, Stearyl alcohol, Myristyl alcohol, Propylene glycol stearate, Titanium dioxide, Palmitic acid, Stearic acid, Dimethicone, Carbomer, Steareth-21, Steareth-2, Disodium EDTA, Sodium hydroxide, Aluminim hydroxide, Phenoxyethanol, Imidazolidinyl urea, Methylparaben, Propylparaben, Benzyl alcohol, Parfum, Hexyl cinnamal, Linalool, Hydroxyisohexyl 3-cyclohexene carboxaldehyde, Butylphenol methylpropional, Alpha-isomethyl ionone, Hydroxycitronellal, Geraniol, Citronellol, Limonene.

Compatability check list

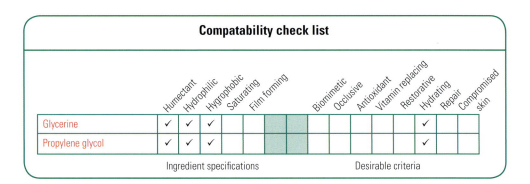

	Humectant	Hydrophilic	Hygrophobic	Saturating	Film forming		Biomimetic	Occlusive	Antioxidant	Vitamin replacing	Restorative	Hydrating	Repair	Compromised skin
Glycerine	✓	✓	✓									✓		
Propylene glycol	✓	✓	✓									✓		

Ingredient specifications   Desirable criteria

Emollients-Saturation-Hydration

Emollients serve two functions: they prevent dryness and protect the skin by acting as a barrier and healing agent, as well as soothing and softening the skin. They reduce roughness; cracking and irritation by temporarily replacing the first line of skin barrier defence "the acid mantle".

Emollients slow TEWL (Trans epidermal water loss)

In addition to their lubricating action, these substances slow TEWL by occlusion thus reducing evaporation of water from the skin surface. In doing so, they induce further hydration of the stratum corneum by the retention of water transported from underlying tissues.

Occlusion works by slowing trans-epidermal water loss (TEWL) and raising hydration levels. The use of occlusive materials, whose action is virtually independent of the environmental humidity, can achieve better hydration through conserving the skin's own water and preventing water evaporation.

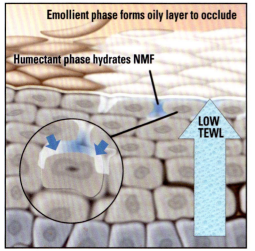

Emollient phase forms oily layer to occlude

Humectant phase hydrates NMF

LOW TEWL

Emollients, often termed skin conditioners, night creams or w/o emulsions, were once based on bland, fatty substances that rendered skin softer and more pliable, however with better refinement methods, emollients that have more affinity with skin lipids are now being used. Examples are rice bran, olive and lecithin oils. With the use of emollients, the stratum corneum will retain its moisture for longer periods of time, resulting in higher extensibility and a less lipid dry appearance. Although virtually any fatty material can make the skin feel softer, different emollient agents exert their lubricant actions for differing periods of time, and will consequently produce a variety of different sensations.

Emollients include a very wide range of compounds, ranging from petroleum and related hydrocarbon mineral oils, to relatively non-greasy esters such as isopropyl myristate/ palmitate. Between the extremes lies a large assortment of fats, oils, and waxes including lanolin, fatty acids, fatty alcohols, triglyceride esters, wax esters, and esters of polyhydric alcohols.

Emollient-based creams are composed of water in oil emulsions (w/o); with oil as the largest component which ranges from 3-25%. The concentration of oil in emollient creams is important for easier spreading and the degree of occlusion that is desired.

Emollients fall in to three "weight" categories known as spreading values (SV), with the higher the SV, the firmer (more solid) the substance.

Low spreading value	Medium spreading value	High spreading value
Emollients with low SV are used most often for day & night creams, and around eye products.	Emollients with medium SV most often used in day and sun protection creams and oils.	Emollients with high SV are used in body lotions, hand creams and bath products.
Examples: Castor oil Almond oil Oleyl oleate Rice bran oil	**Examples:** Octyl dodecanol Hexyl decanol Oleyl alcohol Decyl oleate.	**Examples:** Isopropyl stearate Isopropyl palmitate Isopropyl myristate Hexyl laureate

Controversial emollients

Lanolin and it's comedogenic elements

Lanolin was one of the first substances to be employed in an occlusive system, its use as a barrier has been known for thousands of years. Similar to other chemicals, lanolin functionality was thought to be occlusive (preventing the loss of water). Lanolin is a mildly comedogenic substance found in a variety of cosmetic products, and considered a wax rather than a fat.
Lanolin oil is a fluid fraction of lanolin and is also considered mildly comedogenic, with lanolin alcohols ranging from minimally comedogenic to non-comedogenic, when diluted to 10% or less.

The offending comedogenic element of lanolin is lanolic acid. The following derivatives of lanolic acid are considered aggravating to active, oily and acneic skin.

- Isopropyl lanolate   - Hydrogenated lanolin   - Acetylated lanolin alcohol

Hydrocarbons

Hydrocarbons are used in the cosmetic industry quite extensively as lubricants and emollients in lipsticks and creams. These types of cosmetic ingredient are widely used because they are less expensive than others with the same properties.
The level of refinement of these controversial (by some standards) base ingredients will also dictate the price of the end product and its usage. Petrolatum and mineral oil are the two most recognised and historically used hydrocarbons, however there are more modern ingredients such as the aliphatic branched chain hydrocarbons or isoparaffins such as Permethyl® being used that is helping remove the "hydrocarbon" stigma.
Higher end products that are used on the face would demand a very high level of refinement of any hydrocarbon based emollients used, more so than products like hand or body creams. Lower levels of refinement would usually result in a level of contamination and raise the comedogenic and sensitising factors of the end product.

Mineral oil: the most common hydrocarbon in cosmetics

As the name suggests, mineral oil is derived from petroleum, and cosmetic manufacturers use it because it is colourless, odourless, tasteless, very inexpensive, and readily binds other cosmetic ingredients into a smooth, creamy lotion. It is used primarily as a solvent, and the high quality oils used in cosmetics are minimally comedogenic and have low irritancy.

There is sometimes debate (and misinformation) over the use of mineral oil in cosmetics, and it must be understood that all mineral oils are not the same, with lower grade oils not of the purity required for skin applications. Cosmetic grade mineral oil is, however the purest form without contaminants and virtually no comedogenic properties.
Quality manufacturers only purchase top-grade products from reputable suppliers who guarantee the standards of the materials they provide, and this will be reflected in the price of the formulation, and end user product.

Common hydrocarbons used as emollients:

- Petroleum distillate
- Petrolatum
- Isoparaffin C9-11

- Polyethylene
- Mineral oil
- Isoparaffin C11-13

- Polybutene
- Isoparaffin c8-9
- Isoparaffin C13-16

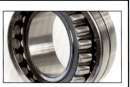

40LD: $19.20
(Industrial use)

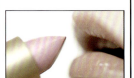

70FG: $90.45
(Cosmetic use)

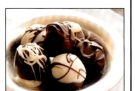

500FG: $114.70
(Food use)

High grade oils:
price per 20 litres $USD

Silicone as an emollient

Just like hydrocarbons, silicones can form polymers, and so are used as emollients, lubricants, thickeners and coatings, to help substances feel smooth.
In cosmetics and personal care products, there are two families of unmodified silicones widely used; dimethicones (also known as polydimethylsiloxane or PDMS) and cyclomethicones (also known as decamethylcyclo-pentasiloxane). These silicone compounds are particularly known for unusual flowing and non-flammable properties and optical clarity as well as being inert and non-toxic. They are also used as an emulsifier for "water-in-oil" emulsions.

Common silicone and methicone based compounds used in cosmetics include:

- Amino bispropyl dimethicone
- Amodimethicone
- Behenoxy dimethicone
- C24-28 alkyl dimethicone
- Cetearyl methicone
- Dimethoxysilyl ethylenediaminopropyl dimethicone
- Hydroxypropyldimethicone
- Stearoxy dimethicone
- Stearyl dimethicone

- Aminopropyl dimethicone
- Amodimethicone hydroxystearate
- Cyclopentasiloxane
- C30-45 alkyl methicone
- Cetyl dimethicone
- Hexyl methicone
- Stearamidopropyl dimethicone
- Stearyl methicone
- Vinyl dimethicone

Film formers as emollients

You will be familiar with substances such as hyaluronic acid (sodium hyaluronate) having film forming and saturating abilities when applied to the stratum corneum. There are however, many other types of chemicals that have the same film forming properties.
Many of these blends are distributed under trade names as compounds or special active ingredients, and are mostly found in sun protection products, moisturisers and lipsticks.

The table below shows common film formers and their respective properties.

Film forming emollients	Examples of use
Brassica campestris / Aleurites fordi oil copolymer	Film-forming, occlusive polymer for emulsions
Hydrogenated polyisobutene	Water-proofing properties for emulsions
Polyisobutene isoparaffin	Highly occlusive and film forming, high viscosity
Polyisobutene (and) C18-21 alkane	Film formation, improves barrier properties
Polyisobutene (and) C12-14 isoparaffin (and) C15-19 alkane	Film former, water-resistance & shine
Polyquaternium-4	Conditioner, film-former

Fatty acids (FFAs)

Skin surface lipids and skin barrier defence differences are reflected in the quality and quantity of the acid mantle lipids, and these are often determined by age, sex, living /working environment and temperatures/humidity. A typical acid mantle skin lipid composition is shown below, and by understanding more about the types of lipids that make up an acid mantle, a skin clinician should be able to put together a treatment program or choose products that would mimic this invaluable first line of skin barrier defence.

When looking at the composition of a typical acid mantle you will notice that the highest percentage of the lipids are triglycerides 30%, waxes 27% and fatty acids 24%.

All of these lipids are commonly used in the emollient phase of a cream, and the whole acid mantle composition is very much like a w/o based cream or a night cream. Both are occlusive and effectively slow TEWL.

Typical composition of skin surface lipids

- Triglycerides   30%   • Waxes   27%
- Fatty acids   24%   • Squalene   12%
- Cholesterol esters   3%   • Diglycerides   2%
- Cholesterol   1%   • Ceramides & glucoceramides 1%

Triglycerides are the main constituents of vegetable oils and animal fats. Triglycerides have lower densities than water (they float on water), and at normal room temperatures they may be solid or liquid. When solid, they are called "fats" or "butters" and when liquid they are called "oils".

A triglyceride, is a chemical compound formed from one molecule of glycerol and three fatty acids. We know that up to 30% of skin surface lipids (the acid mantle) are triglycerides, therefore when some of those important saturated fats are missing, skin will suffer.

Free fatty acids

Free fatty acids are also an important part of the acid mantle, playing the role in ensuring that a constant 5.5 pH is maintained. Free fatty acids are also widely used in cosmetic formulations primarily as emollients and emulsifiers, as they are very suitable in products for skins that are very lipid dry or have an impaired acid mantle. However, over the years, it has been found that some FFAs are too emollient and have a comedogenic effect on active oily skins, so formulators must be mindful when preparing a product designed for this skin type and related skin conditions.

Oily skins generally have an abundance of FFAs as part of the acid mantle, and when products that contain large percentages of FFAs (example: oleic acid) such as moisturisers and foundations are applied and left on the skin surface, comedones and pustules are often the result.

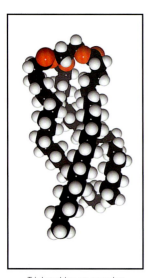

Triglycerides are complex molecular structures comprised of one molecule of glycerol and three fatty acids

Comedogenicity

Some substances are found to be only minimally comedogenic whilst others are severely comedogenic.
Refer to comedogenic scale on page 40 for more details.

Major fatty acids found in the acid mantle			
Palmitic acid	25.3%	Cis-Hexadecc-6enoic	21.7%
Pentadecanoic	4.0%	Cis-14-Methylpentadec-6-enoic	4.0%
Stearic	2.9%	Myristic	6.9%
Cis-Octadec-6-enoic (Petroselenic)	1.9%	cis0Octadec-8-enoic	8.8%
Oleic	1.9%		

Oleic acid: monounsaturated and poly saturated oil (omega 9 / n-9)

Unlike alpha-linolenic acid (n-3) and linoleic acid (n-6) fatty acids, oleic acid (n–9) fatty acids are not classed as essential fatty acids; (EFAs) this is because they can be metabolised by the human body from the omega 3 and omega 6 unsaturated fats, and are therefore not essential in the diet.
It is now considered that many of us have an over-abundance of omega 6 & 9 (Linoleic acid and oleic acid) in our diets.
Some n–9s are common components of animal fat and vegetable oil. The two n–9 fatty acids important in industry are: oleic acid (18:1, n–9), which is a main component of olive oil and other monounsaturated fats, and erucic acid (22:1, n–9), which is found in rapeseed, wallflower seed, and mustard seed.
Oleic acid oil makes up 55% to 80% olive oil, though there may be only 0.5 – 2.5% or so as actual free acid and 15 – 20% of grape seed oil and sea buckthorn oil. The Brazilian palmberry, acai, contains one of the highest concentrations of oleic acid, (56%) which is found in the pulp of the fruit.
There are many fatty acids that make up triglycerides and diglycerides. They are listed below for easy reference and grouped from saturated through to monounsaturated and polyunsaturated to help you choose an oil for the benefits they can bring to skin, including compatibility to skin lipids.

Percent by weight of total fatty acids									
Oil or Fat Type	**U/S Ratio**	**Saturated**					**Mono**	**Poly**	
	Unsat./ Sat.ratio	Capric acid C10:0	Lauric acid C12:0	Myristic acid C14:0	Palmitic acid C16:0	Stearic acid C18:0	Oleic acid C18:1	Linoleic acid (6) C18:2	Alpha-linolenic acid (3) C18:3
Almond oil	9.7	-	-	-	7	2	69	17	-
Canola oil	15.7	-	-	-	4	2	62	22	10
Cocoa butter	0.6	-	-	-	25	38	32	3	-
Cod liver oil	2.9	-	-	8	17	-	22	5	-
Coconut oil	0.1	6	47	18	9	3	6	2	-
Corn oil (Maize oil)	6.7	-	-	-	11	2	28	58	1
Cottonseed oil	2.8	-	-	1	22	3	19	54	1
Flaxseed oil	9.0	-	-	-	3	7	21	16	53
Grape seed oil	7.3	-	-	-	8	4	15	73	-
Illipe oil	0.6	-	-	-	17	45	35	1	-
Olive oil	4.6	-	-	-	13	3	71	10	1
Palm oil	1.0	-	-	1	45	4	40	10	-
Palm olein	1.3	-	-	1	37	4	46	11	-
Palm kernel oil	0.2	4	48	16	8	3	15	2	-
Peanut oil	4.0	-	-	-	11	2	48	32	-
Safflower oil	10.1	-	-	-	7	2	13	78	-
Sesame oil	6.6	-	-	-	9	4	41	45	-
Shea nut oil	1.1	-	1	-	4	39	44	5	-
Soybean oil	5.7	-	-	-	11	4	24	54	7
Sunflower il	7.3	-	-	-	7	5	19	68	1
Walnut oil	5.3	-	-	-	11	5	28	51	5

Emollients that mimic skin structure & function

Omega 9: not an EFA

These monounsaturated fats are not classified as essential fatty acids (EFAs) because they can be metabolised from omega's 3 and 6.

It should be noted that some marketers of products containing omega 9's still promote them as EFAs despite it being chemically incorrect. This may be due to either ignorance or to purposefully mislead.

Essential fatty acids

Essential fatty acids (EFAs) consist principally of unsaturated linoleic, alpha-linolenic and arachidonic acid and form the basic building blocks of body fats, biological membranes and prostaglandins.
They are more commonly recognised by their "omega" names: omega 3, omega 6 and historically this omega group were known as vitamin F.
EFA's are not metabolised by the body, (except omega 9) and the only source is via diet or topical application. With this in mind, EFAs should be a critical constituent of any ingested oils, as well as an active emollient within a creams formulation, as it is required for optimum maintenance of the cutaneous barrier function. Essential fatty acids are a special group of oils with great affinity to epidermic lipids and cellular membranes, with all the therapeutic qualities that treat eczema, dermatitis, lipid dryness, itchyosis and of course, essential fatty acid deficiency.

Any deficiency of the EFAs will lead to compromised cell membranes, oxidative stress and lipid peroxidation. EFAD will also cause a reduction in the formation of prostaglandins, the most important to skin cells being prostaglandin 3, which will result in cellular inflammation.

The cell membrane consists of three classes of amphipathic lipids: phospholipids, glycolipids, and steroids. The amount of each depends upon the type of cell, but in the majority of cases, phospholipids are the most abundant of those cells in the epidermis. For these phospholipids to remain lipophilic and viable, it has been found that 4% percent essential fatty acids such as linoleic acid and alpha linolenic acid are essential.

Essential fatty acids in cosmetic formulations

It has been established that polyunsaturated vegetable phospholipids containing linoleic and alpha-linolenic acids increase the permeability of the cell membranes and improve all skin barrier defence systems.
Topically applied EFAs are easily metabolised from surface application and formulators find them easy to incorporate into cosmetic formulations, making them a more attractive choice.
Omegas come from both plant and marine sources and the continuing interest by skin care formulators means that acceptance, as an important skin treatment active is strong. Omegas 3 and 6 are leaders in the new formulations of today, playing major roles in the creation of "emulsifier free" formulations that bio-mimic skin structure and function.

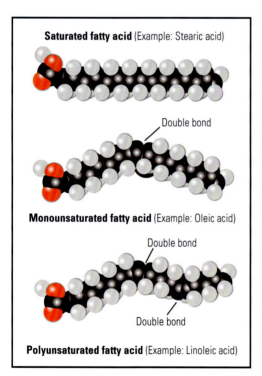

Saturated fatty acid (Example: Stearic acid)

Double bond

Monounsaturated fatty acid (Example: Oleic acid)

Double bond

Double bond

Polyunsaturated fatty acid (Example: Linoleic acid)

The molecular differences between unsaturated and saturated fats. The double bond causes the bends.

Kiwi fruit seed oil as a source of alpha linolenic acid

Kiwi oil (from kiwifruit) has a high content of alpha linolenic acid (ALA). It typically contains around 61% ALA which is higher than many of the other conventional oils commercially available. (e.g. flax, camelina, hemp, walnut oil)

Camelina oil as a source of alpha linolenic acid

The golden orange seeds produced by this plant contain around 40% of oil rich in Omega 3 fatty acids. It is an ideal treatment medium for EFAD and cellular inflammation.

Hemp seed oil as a source of alpha linolenic and linoleic acids

Extracted from seed produced from a special variety of hemp seed, this oil is a good natural source of both the essential fatty acids, linoleic acid (Omega 6) and alpha linolenic acid (Omega 3). Hemp has good skin protection properties and is particularly useful in the treatment of lipid dry skin and EFAD.

The chart below provides information on a range of sources of EFAs used in the cosmetic industry and shows the metabolic pathways and some of the other terms for EFAs, for example docosahexaenic acid (DHA) and eicosapentaenoid acid. (EPA)

EFA	Metabolic pathways of Linoleic & Alpha Linolenic acid	Good sources of Omega 3 & Omega 6 for cosmetic formulatory use	Blocking factors	Enhancing factors
Omega 3	Alpha linolenic acid	Hemp seed oil INCI: Cannabis sativa	Ageing	Vitamin B6
			Alcohol	Vitamin C
	Delta 5 Desaturase	Flax seed oil INCI: Linum usitatissimun	Chemical carcinogens	Vitamin E
	Eicosapentaenoid acid (EPA)	Soybean oil INCI: Trisodium phosphate	High cholesterol diet	Zinc
	Docosahexaenic acid (DHA)	Kiwi fruit seed oil INCI: Actinidia chinensis	Diets high in saturated fats	Ceramides
	Prostaglandin 3 (PG3)	Camelina oil: INCI: Camelina Sativa Seed Oil	Diets high in sugar	Liposomes
Omega 6	Linoleic acid	Borage oil INCI: Borago officinalis	Diabetes	Alpha lipoic
	Delta 6 Desaturase	Evening primrose INCI: Oenothera biennis	Low levels of MG or Zn	Magnesium
	Gamma Linolenic acid (GLA)	Spirulina	Low levels of Vit B6 & Vit C.	Selenium
		Sunflower oil INCI: Helianthus annus	Radiation	
	Dihomo-Gamma-Linolenic Acid	Black current oils INCI: Ribes nigrum	Trans-linoleic acids	
	Arachidonic acid	Olive oil INCI: Olea europea	Viral disease	
	Prostaglandin 1 (PGE1)	Safflower oil Binomial name: Carthamus tinctorius	Genetic inability to convert EFA's	
	Prostaglandin 2 (PGE 2)			

Formulation review

The quality and price of a product will also be reflected by the emollients used, and their affinity with the oil soluble phases of the epidermis. (e.g. acid mantle, bilayers, cell membrane)
Reviewing what you have read in this section;

1. Do you believe the emollients used in our example below would have an affinity with the oil phases of the epidermis?

2. Are any of these ingredients comedogenic? (Refer table on page 40)

3. Would this product be suitable for an active oily skin?

4. This product was labelled as an anti-ageing cream. Do any of the emollients listed address skin ageing?

5. Are there any silicones being used as emollients? How many?

6. Do any of these emollients mimic an oil phase of the epidermis?

Ingredients: Aqua, Glycerine, Niacinamide, Cetyl alcohol, Propylene glycol, Petrolatum, Cyclopentasiloxane, Isopropyl palmitate, Panthenol, Tocopherol acetate, Tocopherol, Camellia sinensis, Ceramide 3, Stearyl alcohol, Myristyl alcohol, Propylene glycol stearate, Titanium dioxide, Palmitic acid, Stearic acid, Dimethicone, Carbomer, Steareth-21, Steareth-2, Disodium EDTA, Sodium hydroxide, Aluminim hydroxide, Phenoxyethanol, Imidazolidinyl urea, Methylparaben, Propylparaben, Benzyl alcohol, Parfum, Hexyl cinnamal, Linalool, Hydroxyisohexyl 3-cyclohexene carboxaldehyde, Butylphenol methylpropional, Alpha-isomethyl ionone, Hydroxycitronellal, Geraniol, Citronellol, Limonene.

Compatability check list

	Emollient	Silicone	Free fatty acid	Petroleum base	Film forming		Biomimetic	Occlusive	Antioxidant	Vitamin	Restorative	Hydrating	Repair	Compromised skin
Petrolatum	✔			✔	✔			✔						
Cyclopentasiloxane	✔	✔			✔			✔						
Isopropyl palmitate	✔		✔									✔		
Ceramide 3	✔						✔					✔		✔
Myristyl acohol	✔		✔											
Propylene glycol stearate	✔											✔		
Palmitic acid	✔		✔		✔							✔		✔
Dimethicone	✔	✔			✔			✔						

Ingredient specifications   Desirable criteria

Cosmetic formulation delivery systems

Consumers expect and demand real performance and benefits from their products. They are educated on the perceivable benefits from certain ingredients and draw parallels between the ingredients and their benefits to the skin.

By creating ingredients that mimic skin functions and cell requirements, formulators are making skin creams that do offer a result. With the advent of these new materials, comes a whole new set of formulating challenges.

These new ingredients can sometimes be unstable, irritating to skin, or difficult to incorporate into cosmetic products, so by encapsulating them into delivery systems that are compatible with surrounding cells, the risk of rejection is reduced.

Delivery systems and controlled release technology are expanding the cosmetics industry into areas previously known only to pharmaceutical companies. The industry is experiencing a dramatic wave of innovation to address new market driven opportunities. Consumers today are much more sophisticated and educated than in the past, especially in areas of skin care and ageing. This is due to vigorous advertising and marketing campaigns by cosmetic companies.

Controlled release delivery systems

The objective of most controlled release delivery vehicles is to deliver the active ingredients to a specific target site while stabilising those ingredients and maintaining the final product's aesthetics.

This can be accomplished in different ways, with the modulating of the skin barrier function the most effective. This method uses vehicles composed of materials similar to the skin lipid content, allowing increased penetration of materials that would otherwise be unable to penetrate this very selective barrier.

Vehicles can also be designed to adhere to the skin surface to provide benefits to the skin surface, to reinforce or to replace the acid mantle.

Not on the list?

Liposomes are not listed as such on ingredient labels, however the substances forming the "liposome" itself and it's contents (if any) are.
Typically, the combination of ingredients will be listed as a group with "and" between the ingredients instead of a comma.

Example:
...water and alcohol and lecithin and safflower oil and tocopherol acetate.....

Benefits of delivery systems	Specific examples
Overcoming ingredient incompatibilities.	Oil soluble active ingredients can be placed into clear, aqueous systems.
Preventing oxidation or decomposition.	Ingredients subject to oxidation such as vitamin C can be protected from air.
Lengthening shelf life of final products.	Protection from oxidation of specific ingredients, prevents discolouration of finished products.
Improving aesthetics.	Encapsulation of glycerine reduces tack and allows its incorporation into dry powdery systems.
Reducing irritancy of key ingredients.	Encapsulation of AHA's.
Providing continuous benefits instead of a single limited exposure.	Anti-irritants can soothe skin for sustained periods of time instead of a single limited applicaton.

Liposomes

Liposomes are microscopic, fluid-filled spheres whose walls are made of layers of phospholipids which are analogous to the phospholipids that make up cell membranes in our skin.

Liposomes can be custom designed for almost any need by varying the lipid content, size, surface charge and method of preparation, making them suitable for delivery systems for pharmaceuticals, vitamins and cosmetic materials.

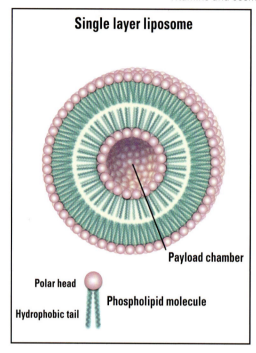

Single layer liposome

Payload chamber

Polar head

Phospholipid molecule

Hydrophobic tail

There are three basic types of liposomes:

- Small unilamellar vesicles: single layer of bimolecular membranes (small uniform size). (SLV or single lamellar vesicle structure)
- Multilamellar: with multiple layers of bi-molecular membranes. (MLV or multi-lamellar vesicle structure)
- Large unilamellar vesicles: single layer of bi-molecular membranes (not uniform in size).

Liposomes obtained from soybean lecithin phospholipids have proven to be the most compatible to the cell membrane, bi-layers and acid mantle.

Liposomes are not moisturisers in the common sense, but biomimic the bilayers of the stratum corneum and cell membrane lipids, helping slow TEWL.

The three phase absorption of liposomes

Upon application, the outer phospholipid shell of the liposome becomes bound superficially to the keratin of the stratum corneum, and this process is responsible for the spontaneous feeling of the skin being coated after application.

As a result of its slightly occlusive effect, the film reduces trans-epidermal water loss, augmenting the barrier function of the skin.

As the liposomes travel through the lipid bi-layers, more of the phospholipids are "melted" into the oil phase of the layers, further supplementing the skin barrier defence systems at the same time. The water phase of the liposome is also being released into the bilayers of the SC, thus improving the saturation of the skin. Concurrently, the encapsulated active payload is being released as the liposome "melts" through the layers of the epidermis.

The remaining phospholipids of the liposomes are introduced into the deeper layers of the skin, assimilating with cell membranes. This explains the potential three-phase effect of the phospholipids in liposome formulations on application to the skin.

Are all liposomes created equal?

Liposome technology has come a long way since the early 90's when the liposomes of the era were very fragile and unstable. Even then, however premium serums had up to 2400 liposomes per drop. Today, numerous liposomes with active compounds already loaded for specific skin conditions are available. The major difference between liposome products today is in what has been loaded into the liposome. This is where the value is, as many domestic retail products use liposomes containing only water.

These "empty" liposomes are often the reason why the products can be of a more modest price.

Empty vessels?

Some supermarket priced cosmetic products utilising liposomes will often feature "empty" liposomes or contain low quality actives within.

The quality and size of the liposomes used will often be drastically different to more professional or therapeutic formulations.

"You get what you pay for"

Nanotechnology

The term nanotechnology refers to structures of the size 100 nanometers or smaller, and involves developing materials or devices within that size. Nanotechnology is not new, in fact it was being discussed over 20 years ago with the micronisation of titanium dioxide and zinc oxide.
There has been much debate on the future implications of nanotechnology, including concerns about potential toxicity of substances that can readily transverse the skin barrier defence systems.

Nanoparticles

The most original types of nanoparticles in personal care, are the attenuating grades of titanium dioxide and zinc oxide. A small particle size is required with these materials to provide transparency on application and cosmetic aesthetics. This does not always equate to full UV protection.
Other organic particles such as nano-scale forms of iron oxide, silica and alumina, also have found application in cosmetic products as make-up colours.
Peptides have already changed the face of the "beauty industry" and the smaller nanomaterials will do the same. The challenge lies in the particle size and if nanos become too small they will be "prescription only," reducing the market considerably. Not such a bad thing if you're an appearance medicine doctor, but this won't work for the large professional beauty and retail personal care industry (which is a bigger market).

There are few benefits to the personal care industry if nanotechnology becomes too small, many actives would greatly benefit skin if they could transverse the skin barrier defence systems and reach a target cell. The question is can an active be selective and only target a specific cell and remain being called a cosmetic? (I don't think so)

Nanosomes

Nanosomes are single or double bilayer structures that are so small they are measured in the nanometer range, (hence the name) and are approximately 800 times smaller (typically 50 nanometers in size) than the diameter of the human hair.
Nanosomes can be up to twenty times smaller than liposomes, dependant on type, and these tiny, liposome-like carriers differ from their larger brothers in both composition and manufacturing process.

Nanosomes are composed from much higher quality phospholipid ingredients than the commercial lecithin from which the larger liposomes are created, some with higher percentages of phosphatidylcholine (PC), an essential component of cell membranes and found in lecithin.
Lecithin, a commonly used source for liposomes typically contains only 10-20% phosphatidylcholine, however higher grades used to create nanosomes may contain up to 40% phosphatidylcholine.

As the higher-grade materials that make up the nanosomes are believed to possess more skin cell compatibles than conventional liposomes, they possess greater non- antigenic properties and are more biodegradable.
Some of the processes to create nanosomes include the use of high-pressure "supercritical fluids" or by subjecting large, multiple-layer liposomes to ultrasonic energy. These processes are complex, lengthy, and extremely delicate. Consequently, the cost to produce nanosomes is more expensive than conventional liposomes.

Nanotechnolgy

There is no official, globally recognised definition of the term: it is accepted that nano-scale substances are smaller than 100nm.

The European cosmetics association, Colipa has called for a common definition of the term 'nanomaterial',
that needs to be agreed upon and then applied with common sense.

Currently, different definitions exist in different parts of the world causing confusion for companies operating in a global marketplace.

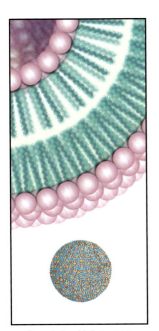

Size relationship between a conventianal liposome and a nanosome

Nanosome advantages

Since nanosomes made with various phospholipid types can contain, encapsulate, and mobilise both water soluble materials as well as oil soluble materials, they can not only deliver a wide variety of encapsulated ingredients to cells, but in the cases of higher grades of materials, also deliver phosphatidylcholine (PC), to help create the cells' own building block.

The PC phospholipid molecule is a universal building block for cell membranes, and the cell's membranes are its essence: they regulate the vast majority of the activities that make up life.

This unique ability of high purity PC nanosomes is claimed to render them potentially one of the most powerful available tools in combating cellular aging.

Due to such small size (the interstices of the outer layer of skin measure about 240 nanometers), nanosomes can more easily penetrate into the skin by topical application, with their active ingredients entrapped inside them, transporting them more efficiently and delivering them to the desired target cells.

Microspheres

Botanical micro-spheres are composed of algae, and their spherical form contains a system of internal canals. The active ingredient is dispersed throughout the sphere in the canals. Release of the active occurs by diffusion from the sphere or by breaking the sphere as it is applied to the skin. In addition to the typical benefits of encapsulation this delivery vehicle has aesthetic appeal for the final cosmetic product. The particles can be large enough to be seen or felt in a cosmetic product, and can even be coloured to achieve a pleasing visual effect.

Micro-sponge®

Micro-sponges® are designed by cross linking monomers into emulsion polymers and then wrapping those polymers into porous bundles.

These systems are typically spherical in shape, ranging in size from one micron to several hundred microns. Their pore sizes range from 0.5 cc/gm to 5 cc/gm. These porous surfaces distinguish Micro-sponges® from traditional liposome type molecules in that Micro-sponges® have many tiny compartments, while liposomes completely enclose active ingredients in a shell-like environment. The highly compartmentalised nature of these materials lends to them a very high internal surface area. This unique feature allows the sponges to function in two very different ways, they can either deliver products by releasing entrapped ingredients, or absorb undesired substances such as excess oil from the skin.

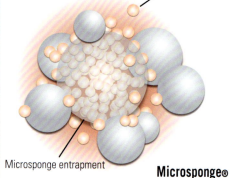

Microsphere

Wall thickness ~ 1um

Active ingredient

Interconnected pores

50 um

Active ingredient

Microsponge entrapment

Microsponge®

Vitamin E based delivery system (tocopherol phosphate mixture)

A new and exciting vitamin E based delivery system has been developed for use in topically applied pharmaceutical products by an Australian bio-technology company (Phosphagenics). Adding a phosphate group to standard vitamin E, was the key to making the ingredient more soluble and stable. The phosphorylated vitamin E is soluble in both oil and water (amphiphilic). As the skin has both lipid and aqueous phases this amphiphilic quality can help the molecule diffuse through the skin more efficiently and encourages the formation of small vesicles, which can be used to transport other ingredients.

This type of delivery system is easily adapted to the cosmetic industry and can be marketed as a carrier, antioxidant and also be cell membrane compatible. This is an ingredient of the new millennium; with compatibility with skin structure and function with an almost "natural" overtone.

Peptides and amino acids

Put simply, peptides are large molecules (sometimes called macromolecules) consisting of linked amino acids. Short bonds, or links between the amino acids are known as peptide, or amide bonds. All proteins in the body (including collagen), consist of amino acids arranged in a linear chain and folded into a globular form, joined by peptide bonds. A protein consists of around 50 or more amino acids and is termed a polypeptide, although the same term is used for a single, linear chain of amino acids.

The difference between polypeptides and peptides is the number of joins and length of chain of amino acids. Peptides are generally termed as being short, while polypeptides are long.

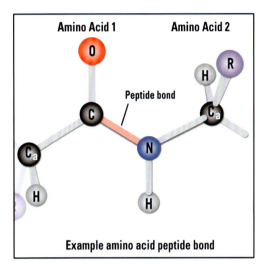

Example amino acid peptide bond

Common types of peptides include:

- Polypeptides are a single, linear chain of amino acids.
- Tripeptides consist of a chain of three amino acids.
- Tetrapeptide has four amino acids.
- Pentapeptides are a chain of five amino acids.
- Oligopeptides refer to chains of between 2 and 20 amino acids.
- Lipopeptides are peptides attached to lipids and proteins.

The role of peptides

Peptides are matrikines (extracellular matrix-derived peptides which regulate cell activity) that influence or direct the cells of the body in some way, with different types of peptides influencing different types of cells.

An example is collagen production; in this scenario, when collagen is broken down, short segments of 3 – 5 amino acids form, and these act as a signal to tell the fibroblast that the collagen fibril is due for replacement or repair and to make new collagen.

Peptides in skin care

The peptides used in skin care are synthetic and also communicate with, and direct the skin cells to behave in a certain way, such as producing more collagen. There is debate over penetration efficacy of some synthetic peptides and proteins as their physical size generally exhibits low diffusivity in the skin. Despite this, popularity and effectiveness of peptides in skin care formulations led to much development of designer and patented peptides with one of the most prominent being palmitoyl pentapeptide-3, which was more commonly known by it's brand name ***Matrixyl®*** .

The current version of ***Matrixyl®*** is now known by its current INCI Name: Glycerine (and) Water (Aqua) (and) Butylene glycol (and) Carbomer (and) Polysorbate 20 (and) Palmitoyl pentapeptide-4. The five peptide sequence for Palmitoyl pentapeptide-4 is ***Lysine-Threonine-Threonine-Lysine-Serine*** (combined with a palmitic acid) with a molecular weight of 620 for the amino chain portion.

Kinetin

A signal peptide derived from plants and also known by the chemical name 6-Furfurylaminopurine, that exhibits antioxidant properties when combined with niacinamide. (B3) It has shown reduced erythema, pigmentation and uniform desquamation.

Dual peptide formulation

Another patented peptide that features a two-peptide synergistic combination of tripeptide with the sequence Pal - Gly - His - Lys, and the tetrapeptide with the sequence Pal - Gly - Gln - Pro - Arg is marketed as ***Matrixyl 3000®***.

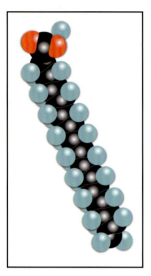

Palmitic acid is a fatty acid that plays a major role in the manufacture of modern cosmetic peptides

Palmitic acid

Also known as hexadecanoic acid, it one of the most common saturated fatty acids found in animals and plants. It is a major component of oil from the palm tree.

When combined with other ingredients, palmitic acid renders them more lipophilic, with greater compatibility with the skin lipids, allowing better penetration.

Palmitoyl

This refers to the palmitoylation or attachment of the fatty acid palmitic acid to the peptide.

Palmitoyl oligopeptide

This synthetic protein is made up of a fragment of collagen and palmitic acid, and is a sequence of six amino acids that reads *valine-glycine-valine-alanine-proline-glycine* combined with a palmitic acid in order to increase penetration through the epidermis. The attachment of palmitic acid is to make the collagen fragment more lipophilic, and more compatible with the skin to allow better penetration.

The research behind this peptide began to help find specific solutions to address ageing factors in the skin, particularly the thinning of the sinusoidal layer between the dermis and the epidermis. The goal was to find a short peptide that would stimulate fibroblasts in the skin to produce key components of the extra-cellular matrix, such as collagen and hyaluronic acid. Palmitoyl oligopeptide can also be found under the trade name of *Biopeptide-CL™*.

Acetyl hexapeptide-3

Also known as *Argireline™*, Acetyl hexapeptide-3 is a hexapeptide (a chain of 6 amino acids) attached to the acetic acid residue. It is believed to work by inhibiting the release of neurotransmitters, and consequently compared to Botox®. However, rather than paralysing facial muscles, these peptides gently relax the muscles by interfering with nerve signals that signal the muscles to contract.

Palmitoyl tetrapeptide-3

Also known under the brand name *Rigin™*, this synthetic peptide is a fragment of immunoglobulin G that has been combined with palmitic acid. This peptide was discovered through research to learn how to suppress the body's production of interleukins, particularly IL6, since these are the chemical messengers that trigger the body's acute inflammatory response.

Palmitoyl tripeptide-3 reportedly works to increase collagen production by mimicking the body's own skin collagen production regulator. The mechanics of this may be to control the L-ascorbic acid, that is an essential cofactor to the lysyl hydroxylase and prolyl hydroxylase enzymes essential for collagen biosynthesis. This peptide is sometimes referred to as *Palmitoyl tetrapeptide-7.*

Copper peptides

Certain kinds of peptides have an avid affinity for copper, to which they bind very tightly. The resulting compound consisting of a peptide and a copper atom has become known as a copper peptide. The mechanism of copper peptide action is relatively complex. The peptide chain of *glycyl-L-histidyl-L-lysine-Cu* induces the degradation of "extra-large" collagen aggregates found in scars and promotes the synthesis of smaller more regular collagen found in normal skin. It also promotes the synthesis of elastin, proteoglycans, glycosaminoglycans and other components of the skin matrix. Other important effects of copper peptide chains include the ability to regulate the growth rate and migration of different types of cells; a significant anti-inflammatory action, and the ability to prevent the release of oxidation-promoting iron into the tissues. The net result is faster, better and "cleaner" healing. The sequence of *glycyl-L-histidyl-L-lysine* is also known as GHK.

Biomimetic peptides

These peptides reduce corneocyte cell to cell adhesion, (desmosomes) improving skin conditions such as hyperkeratinisation and keratosis pilaris. The amino chains in these peptides is hexanol- *Arginine - Alanine - Norleucine.* This peptide was designed for delivery to the corneodesmosomes of the deeper stratum corneum. The *PerfectionPeptide P3* is an example of this technology.

Formulatory processing aids

There are many cosmetic ingredients that fall into this category. Put simply, they are any substances used to assist in the mixing of individual ingredients or impart desirable texture or physical properties to a formulation.

Some of the individual functions of these ingredients have already been mentioned and it is important to remember that many of the substances used as processing aids are multi-functional. This means they will impart different characteristics dependent on the quality and quantity in a formulation.

An example is a substance that can be used as a texturiser in small quantities, and a solvent or lubricant in large quantities. Although most processing aids are non-toxic, some may cause irritation when in high concentrations on specific skin conditions.

Dispersants

A dispersant or a dispersing agent or a plasticiser is either a non-surface active polymer or a surface-active substance added to a suspension (usually a colloid) to improve the separation of particles and to prevent settling or clumping. Dispersants consist normally of one or more surfactants but may also be gases.

Common examples are:

- Alkyl Arylpolyethylene
- Triethanolamine (TEA)
- Glycol Ether
- Polyglycerol ester

Thickeners

Thickening agents such as polymers are often added to cosmetics to change their consistency. Polymers can come from both synthetic sources (eg, polyethylene glycol) or derived from natural sources. (eg, polysaccharides)

Seaweeds are a common source of natural polysaccharides – carrageen is extracted from red algae and alginates from brown algae.

Common thickeners or texturisers include:

- Beeswax
- Carbomer 940
- Cocoamide
- Pentaerythrityl tetrastearate
- Xanthan gum
- Carbomer 941
- Cetyl Palmitate
- Polyethylene
- Stearalkonium bentonite
- Magnesium aluminium silicate
- Microcrystalline wax
- Alkyl acrylate crosspolymer
- Cellulose Gum
- Japan wax
- Polybutane
- Calcium carbonate
- Carnauba
- Ozokenite
- Sodium chloride
- Hydroxypropyl methylcellulose
- PEG-120 Methyl glucose dioleate
- Calcium chloride
- Cetyl alcohol
- Paraffin
- Silica
- Carbomer 934
- Ceresin
- Poloxamer 182

Reducers (solvents)

When a formulation is too viscous for the intended application, solvents are used to reduce the consistency. In the case of a solvent with a complex structure a combination of solvents with properties specific to the different phases of the mixture may be required.

Common solvents for reduction in viscosity include:

- C12-15 Alcohols benzoate
- Isopropyl myristate
- Propylene carbonate
- Butyl acetate
- Isopropyl lanolate
- PPG-5-Ceteth-20
- SD Alcohol 3-A

- Demineralised water
- PPG-3 Myristyl ether
- Dicaprylate/dicaprate
- Cyclomethicone
- Isopropyl palmitate
- Propylene glycol
- Water (Aqua)

- Isopropyl alcohol
- Octyl dodecanol
- SD Alcohol 40
- Ethyl acetate
- Poloxamer 182
- Quaternium-26

Alcohols in formulations

Alcohols, in their many forms, are used in skin care and cosmetic formulations for a variety of purposes, and the presence of these substances in formulations is always the source of discussion concerning their claimed beneficial or adverse properties.

The use of alcohols in cosmetic formulations is too frequently misunderstood, as the popular conception of alcohols is that of solvents that dry and irritate the skin. While this is true in the case of many commercial and industrial alcohols, it is important to understand the particular properties of the different alcohols commonly found in cosmetic products, and the roles they play in the formulations.

Simple Alcohols:
• Ethanol • Denatured alcohol • Ethyl alcohol • Methanol • Isopropyl • SD alcohol.

Simple alcohols

The common simple alcohols found in a wide variety of formulations are generally derived from the fermentation of sugars, starches and other carbohydrates. Their major property is that of an antibacterial/antiseptic, but they are also excellent solvents of fats and lipids, and are consequently used in formulations to help remove excess oil and to prepare the skin for procedures such as chemical peels and medical needling.

Simple alcohols are very thin and water-like; they are very volatile and will therefore evaporate very quickly. This rapid evaporation gives astringents the perception of a "tightening" effect and when applied in sufficient quantities and frequency they may induce dry skin conditions.

Denatured alcohol or SDA alcohols are often marketed as being special and different from other alcohols, but are simply alcohols that have been rendered undrinkable by the addition of a denaturant such as denatonium benzoate. Their other properties are largely unchanged.

Aromatic alcohols

These alcohols are used because of their pleasant aromatic odour, and generally perform the same functions as simple alcohols in a formulation, but with a fragrant aspect. They also act as a preservative due to bacteriostatic properties.

Benzyl alcohol is the most widely used aromatic alcohol in cosmetics, and when isolated from essential oils can be an irritant. This type of alcohol is generally used in concentrations below 3%.

Non-drying alcohols (fatty alcohols)

There is another group of more complex alcohols known as fatty alcohols, which exhibit emollient and occlusive properties when used in cosmetic formulations.

These non-drying alcohols have a more complex molecular structure than simple alcohols and are generally derived from both animal and marine sources or synthesised from chemical substitutes.

In their raw state they generally have a thick, waxy texture, although some are almost solid at room temperature.

These thicker, more substantial substances are used in formulations to achieve a smooth velvety feel; they are usually a major emollient or emulsifying portion of cosmetic formulations with a creamy consistency. Their occlusive properties help trap moisture and slow down the transdermal water flow.

Common fatty alcohols include:

- Caprylic alcohol
- Decyl alcohol
- Myristyl alcohol

- Cetearyl alcohol
- Isostearyl alcohol
- Oleyl alcohol

- Cetyl alcohol
- Lauryl alcohol
- Stearyl alcohol

Some fatty alcohols (Oleyl, Isostearyl, Lauryl) exhibit varying degrees of comedogenicity, and when used in high quantities in formulations, may cause adverse reactions on acne prone skins.

Comedogenic effects of raw cosmetic materials

Measuring comedogenicity

During the 1970's a method of measuring the comedogenic factor of cosmetic ingredients known as the "rabbit ear test" was developed; it helped to explain why around 30% of adult women suffered persistent eruption of acne-like comedones induced by the cosmetics they used.

The test method became the benchmark test procedure of several of the larger cosmetic companies at the time. The "rabbit ear test" produced a measurable scale of comedogenicity, ranging from 1 to 5.

On the comedogenicity scale, grades 1 to 2 are considered non-to mildly comedogenic and grades 3 to 5 are considered significantly comedogenic.

Variations on concentrations obviously affected the results of the tests, but certain strongly comedogenic materials remained severely irritating even when diluted to 5 and 10 %.

The reference chart below was produced by extrapolating data from a number of comedogenic assays of common cosmetic raw materials undertaken by a number of cosmetic companies over a ten year period and is provided as a visual guide to comedogenicity.

Only the materials rated over 2.5 have been shown on the chart, with the most comedogenic at the top. For the sake of clarity, we have grouped the ingredients in blocks of the same rating.

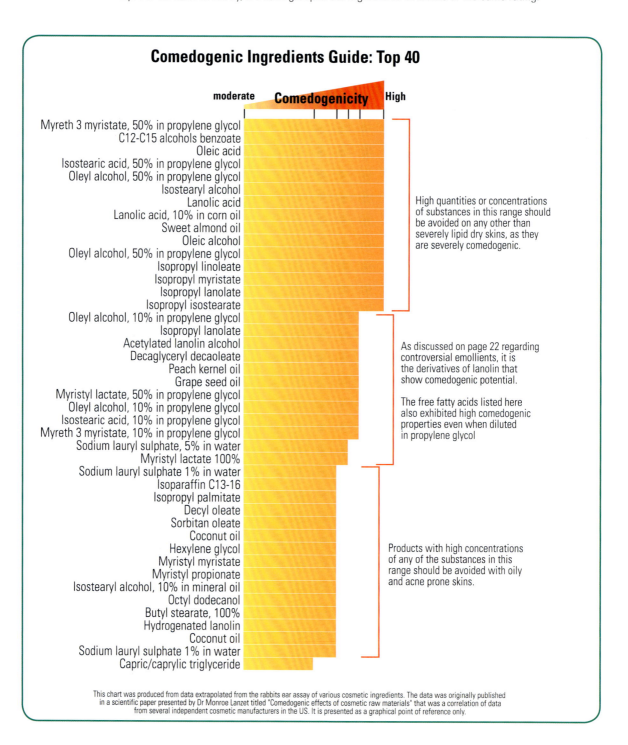

Comedogenic Ingredients Guide: Top 40

moderate — Comedogenicity — High

High quantities or concentrations of substances in this range should be avoided on any other than severely lipid dry skins, as they are severely comedogenic.

As discussed on page 22 regarding controversial emollients, it is the derivatives of lanolin that show comedogenic potential.

The free fatty acids listed here also exhibited high comedogenic properties even when diluted in propylene glycol

Products with high concentrations of any of the substances in this range should be avoided with oily and acne prone skins.

This chart was produced from data extrapolated from the rabbits ear assay of various cosmetic ingredients. The data was originally published in a scientific paper presented by Dr Monroe Lanzet titled "Comedogenic effects of cosmetic raw materials" that was a correlation of data from several independent cosmetic manufacturers in the US. It is presented as a graphical point of reference only.

Formulation review

We have just examined the most common processing aids used in formulations. They are present to provide formulation texture, consistency and "feel nice" properties.

What you will note at this stage of the review process that half the formulation has been surfactants, humectants, emollients and processing aids. Active ingredients are yet to be discovered.

1. Have you come to any conclusions about the quality and price expectation of this cream?

2. Have you found any anti ageing or firming ingredients that would substantiate the marketing claims?

3. Have you identified the fatty alcohols?

4. Have you identified the solvent, texturisers or thickeners?

5. Using the comedogenic table on page 40, can your find any substances that may be a problem for an active oily skin?

Ingredients: Aqua, Glycerine, Niacinamide, Cetyl alcohol, Propylene Glycol, Petrolatum, Cyclopentasiloxane, Isopropyl Palmitate, Panthenol, Tocopherol Acetate, Tocopherol, Camellia Sinensis, Ceramide 3, Stearyl Alcohol, Myristyl Alcohol, Propylene Glycol Stearate, Titanium Dioxide, Palmitic Acid, Stearic Acid, Dimethicone, Carbomer, Steareth-21, Steareth-2, Disodium EDTA, Sodium Hydroxide, Aluminim Hydroxide, Phenoxyethanol, Imidazolidinyl Urea, Methylparaben, Propylparaben, Benzyl Alcohol, Parfum, Hexyl Cinnamal, Linalool, Hydroxyisohexyl 3-Cyclohexene Carboxaldehyde, Butylphenol Methylpropional, Alpha-Isomethyl Ionone, Hydroxycitronellal, Geraniol, Citronellol, Limonene.

Compatability check list

	Solvent	Reagent/catalyst	Texturiser	Thickener	Hygoscopic	Biomimetic	Occlusive	Antioxidant	Vitamin replacing	Restorative	Hydrating	Repair	Compromised skin
Aqua	✓										✓		✓
Carbomer				✓			✓						
Sodium hydroxide		✓			✓								

Ingredient specifications   Desirable criteria

Preservatives

Why preservatives?

A variety of micro-organisms including yeasts, fungi (yeast & mould) and bacteria, including pseudomonas, staphylococci and streptococcus can cause problems with cosmetic preparations over time. Contamination of formulations can lead to separation of emulsions, product discolouration, the formation of gases and odours, as well as the infection of the skin of the user.

Health and safety regulations consequently mandate protection for the consumer. Preservatives are not only in our skin care, make-up and toiletries, but also in our food and medications. We are exposed to preservatives on a wider scale than we would like to think.

Why do products fail?

Problems with preservative failure in cosmetics can be generally related to one or more of the following:

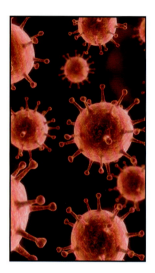

- Expiry of usable shelf life
- Incorrect storage conditions
- Extreme temperature variation during storage
- Incorrect application and usage

Personal care products that usually are stored in bathrooms will contain preservatives to protect against the fungus that inhabit warm damp environments. When one considers the way face creams, masks, eye creams and sun protection are applied and stored then it is easy to understand the need for preservatives. If the end user was as careful about application methods and storage as the clinician is in clinic then the percentage of preservative could be reduced. However this is not the case, and as long as fingers are used to dispense and apply creams, lids are left off containers, products are left unprotected in light and air, there will be a need for preservatives.

Skin conditions most susceptible to preservative reactions

There is a common denominator among skins that show a negative reaction to a product, and most often it is not the product that is at fault. It is generally due to the compromised condition of the skin and would include a loss or reduction in the ***first line of skin barrier defence ,*** the ***"acid mantle".*** The loss of protective "flora" and the emollient and occlusive action of the acid mantle will mean a skin will exhibit the hot, itchy burning signs of eczema and allergic contact dermatitis.

Preservative concerns

The same types of preservatives used in cosmetics are often found in our food and medications. In fact, some may argue that we absorb far more preservatives from these sources than our cosmetics and personal care over any given period of time. Our skin barrier defence systems prevent many preservatives reaching the lower levels of the epidermis, however preservatives in our food and medications are ingested and are more likely to find their way to the bloodstream.

Typical preservatives in our food and medications are:

- Calcium propionate
- BHA (Butylated hydroxyanisole)
- Benzalkonium chloride
- Methyl and propylparaben
- BHT (Butylated hydroxytoluene)
- Disodium EDTA
- Citric acid

Still usable?

It is not uncommon for clients with skin irritations to be unaware that it is the condition of their products that can be the cause of the condition. Clients may be unaware that because of poor storage and useage practices, the product has become "unusable" from a safety standpoint and is harbouring bacteria.

Always check the clients products during the consultation, with particular attention to the state of seals on the packaging and the conditions the products are kept in, and of course the use-by date.

Preservatives in cosmetics are usually only in quantities to protect the formula under normal conditions, however clients can severely test the effectiveness of the preservatives by a combination of poor storage and application habits.

Common preservatives in our skin care and hair products

Each of these common preservatives will protect against a specific microorganism like yeast or mould or a group like gram-positive bacilli, (staphylococcus aureus) or gram negative or sometimes both.

- Paraben family
- DMDM hydantoin
- Benzalkonium chloride
- Dichlorobenzyl alcohol
- Methylisothialinone
- Potassium sorbate
- Sodium dehydroacetate

- Imidazolidinyl urea
- Phenoxyethanol
- Acid ammonium sulphate
- Disodium edetate
- Pentasodium pentetate
- Propyl gallate
- Tetrasodium EDTA (ethylenediaminetetra-acetic acid).

- Quaternium-15
- Benzyl alcohol
- Butylated hydroxytolulene
- Methylchloroisothiazolinone
- Phenoxyethanol
- Sodium benzoate

Preservative compounds

To achieve the broad spectrum of protection required for some commonly used personal care items compounds of preservatives have been developed. This makes a formulation easier to blend and/or to help remove the stigma often attached to some types/names of preservative such as the parabens.

Trade name	INCI name (individual components)
Phenonip	Phenoxyethanol, methylparaben, ethylparaben, butylparaben, propylparaben
Nipaguard POM	Phenoxyethanol (and) piroctone olamine (and) methylparaben
Euxyl K 400	Phenoxyethanol (and) methyldibromoglutaronitrile.
Neolone™ PE	Methylisothiazolinone (and) phenoxyethanol
Neolone™ Cap G	Methylisothiazolinone (and) caprylyl glycol
LiquaGard	Iodopropynyl butylcarbamate in a solvent, butylene glycol.
Bronidox	5-Bromo-5-Nitro-1,3-Dioxane
Nipaguard POB	Phenoxyethanol (and) piroctone olamine (and) benzoic acid
Phenostat	Caprylhydroxamic acid (and) phenoxyethanol (and) methylpropanediol
Botanistat PF64	Phenoxyethanol (and) caprylglycol (and) ethylhexylglycerine (and) hexylene

New frontiers?

The approval for new preservatives is an extremely lengthy, complex and costly process, and consequently there have been no new preservatives approved for use in personal care applications in the EU since 2004.

What you may have noticed in the table above is that other than two compounds, (Phenonip & Nipaguard POM) all of these formulas are "paraben free".

Paraben-free formulations often require the combination of multiple ingredients to effectively preserve a product, and even though globally approved cosmetic preservatives are a rarity today, there are many new options available to formulators.

Some brands will be able to truthfully market as "paraben and formaldehyde free", while others simply disguise their parabens under compound trade names.

Preservatives from the botanical world

All cosmetic formulations require preservatives to protect them from micro-organisms, and there has always been a desire for a more "natural" alternative. Unfortunately, nature does not provide the types of preservatives that are robust enough to survive long-term storage, transportation, temperature extremes and potentially poor application habits.

Suppliers are continually seeking out and developing "natural" preservatives as more and more consumers search for products that are genuinely green and natural. Around the world leading suppliers of cosmetic raw materials have already launched plant-based preservatives that appear to be covering all of the bases as far as being "green and natural", and these are sometimes used alone or in addition to more traditional preservatives. These types of preservatives are filtering through to the skin care industry and it is encouraging to know that alternative botanical based preservatives are here.

An interesting preservative that I have recently been introduced to is under the name of "Plantservative". The name is very appropriate for a "green broad spectrum" (protects against gram positive/gram negative bacteria, yeast and mould). This preservative is derived from the Japanese honeysuckle plant, and according to its developers, is suitable for external cosmetic use.
There are a number of natural organic substances with varying ability to inhibit microbiological growth, and below we have listed three of the most commonly used and respected.

Grapefruit seed extract as a preservative

The holistic community first accepted grapefruit seed extract in the early 90's; from there it has joined a small but effective group of preservatives that carry the label "natural". The Cosmetics Toiletries and Fragrance Association (CTFA) now allow the grape seed extract (GSE) to be printed in their "ingredient recognition" dictionary.
GSE is a broad-spectrum bactericide, fungicide, antiviral and anti-parasitic compound. When used in vitro, GSE has been shown to be highly effective against a broad spectrum of bacteria, including Staphyloccus aureus, Streptococcus pyogenes, Salmonella typhi, Escherichia coli, Pseudomonas aeruginosa, Klebsiella pneumoniae, Shigella dysenteriae, Legionella pneumoniae, Clostridium tetani, Diploccus pneumoniae, and many others.
In the United States, a GSE product called Citricidal® contains 60% grapefruit seed extract in an aqueous, vegetable glycerine solution; and been labelled as GRAS (Generally Recognised as Safe) in the Code of Regulations.

Tea tree oil (Manuka)

Three different species of Tea tree grow in Australia and New Zealand, with the wild New Zealand tea tree commonly known as Manuka (Leptospermum scoparium) and Kanuka (Kunzia ericoides). The Australian tea tree , (Melaleuca alternifolia) is completely different to the New Zealand tea tree, but both of these plants' leaves contain leptospermone, an antibiotic agent.
The oils extracted from tea tree contain 120 elements and can be used medicinally. Manuka oil is well known for its antimicrobial activity, and has been found active against 39 separate micro-organisms. Widely used in the cosmetic, homeopathic, and OTC pharmacy products, Manuka oil can assist in healing and repairing skin and can help to prevent bacterial and fungal growth on the skin surface. Manuka oil is effective against micro organisms, however the concentration required to work as a preservative would need to be unacceptably high, rendering the product toxic and not cosmetically acceptable. When used with other preservatives, lower percentage blends can be utilised.

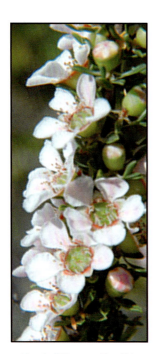

Manuka (NZ tea tree) is widely recognised for its antimicrobial and therapeutic properties

Citric acid as a preservative

Citric acid is also known as the compound 2-hydroxy-1,2,3-propanetricarboxylic acid.
In skin cells citric acid is an intermediary substance in oxidative metabolism, being an important component of the tricarboxylic acid cycle or citric acid cycle and also known as the "Krebs cycle". You may remember as part of your basic aesthetic or beauty therapy training that the "Krebs cycle" is a series of enzyme catalysed chemical reactions of central importance in all living cells that use oxygen as part of cellular respiration.
Citric acid as a stand-alone preservative will not protect against the prevalent micro-organisms but it is widely used throughout the cosmetic industry and it is found in nearly every product on the shelf. Citric acid and its calcium, potassium and sodium salts are used in cosmetics and personal care products to preserve products by chelating (forming bonds) with metals, and to adjust the acid/base balance. Citric acid is a white, crystalline powder that can be extracted from citrus fruits or made from fermented sugar solutions.

Parabens

Parabens are derived from the processing of petroleum and while similar to benzoic acid, are effective at a much higher pH level. Parabens are esters of para-hydroxybenzoic acid, from which the name is derived, and are used primarily for their fungicidal and to a lesser degree their bactericidal properties. In the food industry they are widely found in cheeses, margarines, beverages, pickled products and meats.
Parabens are very active against moulds and yeast, but less effective against bacteria. Given the prevalence of parabens, there are relatively few allergic reactions (typically 3.6% of all adverse reactions) to these substances, and almost all problems occur on skins that have compromised skin barrier defence systems or have a history of allergic contact dermatitis.

Parabens families

The family of parabens involves 4 different types of preservative, with each one protecting from a different bacteria or fungi.

- Methylparaben: anti-fungal (should not be ingested).
- Ethylparaben: commonly found in both food and cosmetics.
- Propylparaben: this anti-fungal is typically found in many water-based cosmetics, such as creams, lotions, shampoos and bath products.
- Butylparaben: anti-fungal.

There are another three lesser used parabens that include isobutylparabens, isopropylparabens and benzylparabens (and their sodium salts).

Paraben controversy

The subject of parabens can raise extremes of opinion regarding safety, and despite the fact that after much study, parabens are not yet officially identified or listed as an endocrine disrupting chemical by any government, medical or regulatory organisation, the classification of parabens by some groups as "toxic" and "cancer causing" continues.
While there are individuals and organisations who genuinely and sincerely believe that parabens are cause for concern, it could be argued that some marketers of "natural" and "preservative free" cosmetic products who foster and support such statements may do so as part of their marketing agenda, rather than a genuine concern. That said, I believe further research as a precautionary principle is necessary to ultimately determine the safety of parabens.

Preservative loophole

In the EU, a marketing "slight of hand" can be used to advertise a product as being "preservative and allergen free" if the preservatives used are not listed in the EU Annex V1, a classification & labelling regulation.

At the time of writing, a preservative that fits into this category is Feniol: INCI: Phenethyl alcohol and Caprylyl Glycol.

Preservative free does not necessarily mean chemical free.....

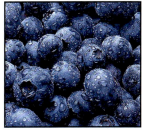

Parabens occur naturally in blueberries, prunes and cinnamon, although all parabens used commercially are made synthetically. In the case of blueberries, the natural presence of methylparaben acts as an antimicrobial agent.

Formaldehyde releasing preservatives

Formaldehyde is an inexpensive and effective preservative that is widely used as a disinfectant, germicide, fungicide and de-foamer. It has been estimated that between 4-8 % of the general population may be sensitised to this popular preservative. More recently, serious questions about the safety of this substance have been raised, to the point that it is prohibited in cosmetics in both Japan and Sweden.

Quaternium-15 (Q-15): A formaldehyde releaser

This is a preservative found in many cosmetics. It is a water-soluble anti-microbial agent that has proven active against bacteria, but less active against yeasts. It was found to be responsible for over 12% of allergic reactions in an American study. It is a formaldehyde releaser, and may be a major cause of dermatitis from preservatives.

People who may be allergic to formaldehyde can potentially have problems with this ingredient. It has also recently been found that quarternum-15 can react in the body with other chemicals to produce nitrosamines (known carcinogens).

Imidazolidinyl urea and diazolidinyl urea

The formaldehyde releaser imidazolidinyl urea is commonly used as a preservative in personal care products and medications. It is active against bacteria, especially pseudomonas species, but it has less activity against fungi. To provide more broad-spectrum activity against gram-positive and gram-negative bacteria and fungi, imidazolidinyl urea is often combined with another preservative such as parabens.

DMDM hydantoin

DMDM hydantoin, another formaldehyde releaser, is one of the most commonly used preservatives in cosmetics today.

It has a broad spectrum of activity against bacteria and fungi, is water-soluble and found most commonly in shampoos, but also in cosmetics.

- 1,3-Dimethylol-5,5-dimethylhydantoin
- 2-Bromo-2-Nitropropane-1,3-diol (Bronopol)

Other sensitising preservatives

Sorbic acid

A common cosmetic preservative that occasionally causes allergic reactions, although it was found to be responsible for only 1.1% of allergic reactions in a study. People allergic to sorbic acid may also react to a related ingredient called potassium sorbate.

Thimerosal

Commonly used in colour cosmetics and mascara, topical medications and some ophthalmic solutions, but not often used in skin care products. It is effective against both bacteria and fungi, however known to cause potential problems with tissue that is already inflamed due to another cause.

Why mixing product lines can cause problems:

It is the knowledge that **Q-15** can react with other chemicals that leads the therapist to the understanding of why it is not good practice to mix brands of cosmetics, or encourage the client to do so.

Cosmetic houses know that the substances within their line are compatible, but generally do not know of the compatibility of their product's preservative with other skin care lines.

Chelating agents

A chelating agent is a chemical that binds to metal ions or other metallic substances in aqueous solutions and inactivates them (reduces their reactivity).

The term "sequestering" metal ions is often used to describe the action of protecting a formulation from metal ions.

Chelating agents are often added to cosmetics to improve the efficiency of preservatives and antioxidants, however they also help form complexes by strengthening chemical bonds, so can be used for multiple purposes. Common chelating ingredients include:

- Disodium EDTA
- Trisodium EDTA
- Tetrasodium EDTA

The suffix EDTA stands for the chemical name ethylenediaminetetraacetic acid.

This group of chemicals will normally be listed in the last two to three lines of a formulation because they are not generally used in large quantities.

Chelating agents come under many other chemical names and it can be difficult to always understand what it is doing in the formulation, so a good rule of thumb is if it is listed with other preservatives at the end of the formulation, it will be likely there as a preservative enhancer, however if it is higher up into the list of ingredients, it may be there as a penetrating enhancer or linked to some other chemical and action.

Minimising the use of preservatives

We know that any cosmetic or personal care product that is truly " preservative free" will usually carry antioxidants as the preservative ingredients. However when a product carries the marketing words "fragrance free" or "preservative free", they will usually have a higher quality and purity of raw materials and the manufacturing plant may or should have practiced what is known as "aseptic manufacturing".

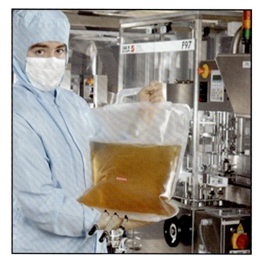

Aseptic manufacturing processes

The term aseptic is defined as preventing infection; free or freed from pathogenic microorganisms; (the methods involved are the most demanding of pharmaceutical manufacturing processes). It requires precise attention to operator training and behaviour, process validation, production process documentation, plant and equipment maintenance and change control management.
Cosmetics claiming the aseptic manufactured certification require the formulations to be manufactured under the most stringent guidelines to prevent any contamination at any time before, during and after the manufacturing process.
The combination of aseptic manufacturing and totally sealed packaging relieves the demand for preservatives, as it minimises the potential for contamination. As you can imagine, adherence to such meticulous processes requires investment in both training and specialised facilities; this has led to some cosmetic brands being manufactured in the same plant as competing brands to maintain quality control with cost effectiveness.

For some smaller cosmetic manufacturers, water conservation, waste minimisation and detoxification regulations may tempt them not to clean and sanitise as frequently, and the only way to compensate for less stringent processes and controls is with higher levels of preservatives.

Specialised packaging

The packaging of "preservative free" cosmetics would ideally be in airtight pump containers. This would ensure that the risk of oxidisation is prevented or reduced. Many ingenious types of packaging have been developed to reduce cross contamination and therefore reduce the need for large quantities of preservatives. With this packaging and controlled storage, spoilage is not as big a problem as it used to be. However once opened, without some form of preservative, damage to the product from air, light and the growth of micro-organisms (e.g., bacteria and fungi) can still occur.

PAO: Period after opening

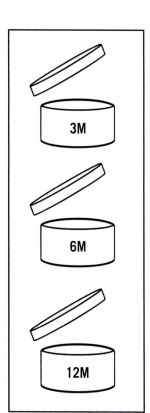

In Europe, there is a specification known as "EU cosmetics directive compliant".
This specification consists of a number of directives with regard to ingredients, preservatives and packaging. This directive specifies labelling of the useable lifespan of cosmetic products, with the Period After Opening (PAO) symbol (shown at left) of an open jar displayed on both the product container and outer packaging.
The lifespan of the product contents in months, is indicated by a number followed by "M".
This can appear either on or next to the open jar symbol.

Cosmetics exempt from the PAO symbol include single use products such as samples and hair dyes, products in packs that have no contact with the air (Aerosols) and very long-lasting products, which do not deteriorate over time.

Formulation review

The formula review now looks at the preservatives in our "anti-ageing" cream.
There are six preservatives, all of which have been mentioned in this segment.

1. Why do you think this formulation requires the number of preservatives/stabilisers highlighted?

2. What component serves a dual purpose?

3. Are there any formaldehyde releasing substances in this group?

4. Which paraben is typically found in water based cosmetic products?

5. What is the name of the paraben found in blueberries?

6. Would this formula be suitable for an ageing, compromised skin?

Ingredients: Aqua, Glycerine, Niacinamide, Cetyl alcohol, Propylene glycol, Petrolatum, Cyclopentasiloxane, Isopropyl palmitate, Panthenol, Tocopherol acetate, Tocopherol, Camellia sinensis, Ceramide 3, Stearyl alcohol, Myristyl alcohol, Propylene glycol stearate, Titanium dioxide, Palmitic acid, Stearic acid, Dimethicone, Carbomer, Steareth-21, Steareth-2, Disodium EDTA, Sodium hydroxide, Aluminim hydroxide, Phenoxyethanol, Imidazolidinyl urea, Methylparaben, Propylparaben, Benzyl alcohol, Parfum, Hexyl cinnamal, Linalool, Hydroxyisohexyl 3-cyclohexene carboxaldehyde, Butylphenol methylpropional, Alpha-isomethyl ionone, Hydroxycitronellal, Geraniol, Citronellol, Limonene.

Compatability check list

	Preservative	Formaldehyde	Chelating	Paraben	Anti-fungal	Anti-microbial	Bactericide	Biomimetic	Occlusive	Antioxidant	Vitamin replacing	Restorative	Hydrating	Repair	Compromised skin
Disodium EDTA	✓		✓												
Phenoxyethanol	✓					✓									
Imidazolidinyl urea	✓	✓					✓								
Methylparaben	✓			✓	✓										
Propylparaben	✓			✓	✓										

Ingredient specifications   Desirable criteria

Fragrance in Formulations

For the skin treatment therapist, awareness of the fragrances used in skin care formulations and the potential issues they can cause is vital. Fragrances are complex substances, and potentially one of the most irritation causative agents of all cosmetic ingredients. Fragrance is also a complex subject because of the secrecy and competition that surrounds it.

One perfume may contain hundreds of different chemicals and the fragrance industry is very competitive. If a company has had a successful fragrance for many years, it is unlikely that they will disclose the chemicals it uses. There are more than 2,800 fragrance ingredients listed in the database of the Research Institute for Fragrance Materials Inc, (RIFM) with at least 100 of these ingredients known as allergens.

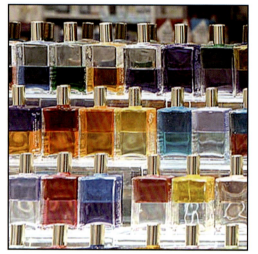

Why fragrance?

If fragrance can cause so many irritation/allergy problems, why include it in cosmetic formulations? There are three primary and obvious reasons for using fragrance in cosmetics:

- To mask the base odour.
- To help support product claims.
- To make the product more aesthetically pleasing.

It should be noted that the use of higher grade of purity in base ingredients will reduce their odour intensity. As a consequence, products manufactured with lower grade raw materials will generally require more fragrance to mask unpleasant odours, and are likely to be more sensitising.

Many of the ingredients contained in skin care products have an inherent odour. These include materials such as lanolin, alcohol, animal and vegetable proteins, vegetable oils and some natural extracts. When these ingredients are blended to make a completed product, the resulting base odour may be unpleasant and render the product unappealing. Fragrances are created to blend with, and mask these base odours, to produce a product much more pleasing to use. Fragrance is an integral part of cosmetic formulations, and it is here to stay. Its use is however regulated to ensure only approved ingredients are employed in formulations.

Regulation of fragrance ingredients

The fragrance industry is self-regulated. This is largely accomplished by a close relationship between the Research Institute for Fragrance Materials (RIFM) and the International Fragrance Association (IFRA). IFRA's Code of Practice currently contains over 100 IFRA standards for fragrance ingredients: about 40 standards prohibiting certain fragrances and about 65 others putting various limitations on their use.

This information is available on the IFRA Web site. (www.ifraorg.org)

Recently, the European Union (EU) designated 26 fragrance allergens as requiring labelling on cosmetic and detergent products.

This labelling must occur if the concentration of the designated ingredient exceeds 100 parts per million (ppm) for a rinse-off product and 10 parts per million (ppm) for a leave-on product.

International Nomenclature of Cosmetic Ingredients (INCI) names must be used.

Introducing "the fragrance mix"

In the late 70's Dr. Walter G Larsen published an article describing the results of his series of tests performed on 20 patients for allergy to fragrance. Dr. Larsen originally used a combination of 30 chemicals in his early series of tests; these 30 chemicals became the basis of the composition of the fragrance mix that has been used internationally ever since to diagnose fragrance allergic patients. "Fragrance Mix 1" was joined by "Fragrance Mix 2" in 2005, and both are used as a point of reference for patch testing for Fragrance Allergy.

The eight ingredients of fragrance mix 1 (all at 1% concentration) are as follows:

- Isoeugenol
- Hydroxycitronellal
- Amyl cinnamal
- Eugenol
- Geraniol
- Evernia prunastri (oak moss) extract
- Cinnamal
- Cinnamyl alcohol

The new fragrance mix 2 constituents are as follows:

- Citronellol 0.5%
- Coumarin 2.5%
- Hydroxyisohexyl 3-cyclohexene carboxaldehyde (Lyral) 2.5%
- Citral 1.0%
- Farnesol 2.5%

Relevance of positive reactions to fragrance mix patch tests

Reactions to individual ingredients of these mixes often only showed frequent irritancy, and low-grade positive reactions, not allergic contact dermatitis. Allergy (allergic contact dermatitis or ACD) is a disease whereas a positive patch-test result is an allergic reaction. One may be allergic, but seldom develop allergic contact dermatitis. This misinterpretation and imprecise language has led clinicians and clients to believe that fragrance allergy (clinical ACD) is much more common than it really is.

Most fragrance is synthetic

Up to 95% of chemicals used in fragrances are synthetic compounds derived from petroleum and coal tar. These include VOCs (volatile organic compounds) such as benzene derivatives, aldehydes, ketones, alcohol denaturants and other known toxins and sensitizers. A study of 31 common fragranced products found 20 shared chemicals between them. They are listed below:

- Ethanol
- Acetone
- B-phenethyl alcohol
- 1-8-cineole
- Benzyl alcohol
- Camphor
- B-citronellol
- A-pinene
- Linalool
- Y-terpinene
- B- benzyl acetate
- Nerol
- A-terpineol
- Methylene chloride
- Limonene
- Ethyl Acetate
- B-myrcene
- A-terpinolene
- Benzaldehyde
- Ocimene

Fragrance fixing agents

In perfumery, a fixative is a natural or synthetic substance used to reduce the evaporation rate and improve stability when added to more volatile components. This allows the final product to last longer while keeping its original fragrance. Fixatives are indispensable commodities to the perfume industry. Some examples of fixatives are sandlewood, musk, vetiver, and orris root. Natural fixatives usually have a fragrance that is considered a "base note" in perfumery terms, reflecting their low volatility.

Fragrance in marketing and product perception

Marketing companies have over the years used fragrance and colour to help support the perceived claims of their products. Product image provides a guideline for the fragrance chosen, while supporting any special attributes and therapeutic properties.
Some examples of how fragrance and colour are used in synergy:

- Lower levels of a soft floral blend for example, can enhance the perception of greater smoothing and moisturising properties.
- The use of green, light floral ozone and or citrus notes in a fragrance will enhance the consumers' perception of refreshing natural skin toning.
- Mint fragrances with a hint of green colour usually indicate something suitable for an oily or problem skin.
- A soft rose fragrance and pink colouring is often used for a mature dry skin.

Essential oils as fragrance

Fragrant emollient esters, such as essential oils, have been used as fragrance in cosmetic preparations for centuries. Beside their fragrance they also have additional properties. (Refer page 58 for more detail on essential oils)

Fragrance free, hypoallergenic and other ambiguities

Marketing terms such as hypoallergenic, dermatology tested, allergy screened and fragrance free can, at best, be vague and unspecific.
The labelling of "fragrance fee" may only mean that a product has less fragrance than a fragranced version of the same product from that manufacturer, and some countries allow scent-free labelling on products that contain .06% or less of fragrance. Others use the term "masking agent" when fragrance is used in small quantities.
The term hypoallergenic has no medical definition, and there are no industry standards of measurement and legal definition of any of these commonly used statements. Consequently, until they are defined, they are open to individual interpretation and marketing abuse.

Colour in formulations

Deciphering packaging disclosure

Even high profile and expensive domestic retail products can contain ingredients, fragrances and colourings that may not always come from the best source.

The belief that price or labelling stating "for beauty therapy or professional use only" will ensure a higher quality or refinement of ingredients is no guarantee in the case of colour cosmetics (make-up) and colours used in cosmetics.

With the advent of product composition disclosure on packaging, the task of finding out what colourings are present is now far easier. What is still difficult is deciphering the international packaging and labelling laws; each country and or state having differences of opinion on what is "safe" when it comes to colour used in cosmetics.

The EU has a list of approved colours, as does the US and Japan, the number of colours common to all is relatively small. This lack of harmonisation means that industry cannot sell products across all markets. In some cases, test methods, formulation, packaging and advertising requirements differ.

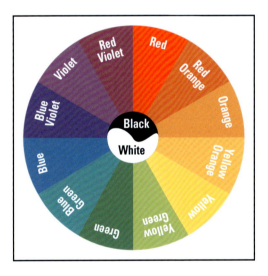

F D & C colours

American regulations provide for colours used in food, drugs and cosmetics to be listed under the prefix of F D & C Colours. This prefix is perhaps the most widely known because of its use in the naming of food colouring additives. There is also a group of some colourings that are classified as being generally recognised as safe (GRAS) by the FDA and do not require certification.

Colours used in food, drugs and cosmetics are classified by type with a letter code (F, D, or C), which indicates the use for which it is approved. These letters will precede the number and description of the colour. An example is F D&C yellow No5.

- When F D&C precede a colour it means the colour can be used in food, drugs or cosmetics.
- D&C signify that it can only be used in drugs and cosmetics, and not in food.
- Ext D& C before a colour means that it is certified for use in drugs and cosmetics for external use only, and may not be used on the lips or mucous membranes.

I have used the FDA colour classification as my point of reference, although many of us are in countries that use other colour classifications such as the EU, who use the letter "E" as a suffix to a number identifying colours, preservatives and other regulated ingredients. It was the lack of agreement between countries regarding standards for colourings that made writing this component in generic manner a challenge.

The FDA lists only nine colour additives that can be used in all three classifications of food, drugs & cosmetics (FD&C). There are many colours approved for the use in drugs and cosmetics (D&C) only, which is interesting because one would have thought that drugs (pharmaceutical) and cosmetics were as important as food, and as frequently used (drugs if not more so).

The colour story is huge, and I decided not too get to in-depth, suffice to say that there is an enormous amount of information on the internet, and I suggest you use government or health authority run web sites for what would be classified as the most updated industry information that all formulators use. I have included with the table on the following page (created from information found on Wikipedia) the European Union colour classification number when it was available.

FDA Certifiable Colors for use in food, drugs and cosmetics (FD&C)				
FDA name	**EU No**	**Common name**	**Colour**	**Comments**
FD&C Blue No. 1	E133	Brilliant Blue FCF	Bright blue	A synthetic dye derived from coal tar. It can be combined with tartrazine (lemon yellow azo dye E102) to produce various shades of green.
FD&C Blue No. 2	E132	Indigotine	Royal blue (blue jeans)	Indigo dye is an organic compound with a distinctive blue colour. Historically, indigo was extracted from plants, and was rare. Almost all indigo produced today is synthetic.
FD&C Green No. 3	E143	Fast Green FCF	Sea green	A sea green triarylmethane food dye that is used for tinned green peas and other vegetables, jellies sauces, fish, desserts and dry bakery mixes at level of up to 100 mg/kg. It is prohibited in the EU and some other countries for use as a food dye.
FD&C Red No. 3	E127	Erythrosine	Cherry red	Used as a food colouring, in printing inks, as a biological stain, a dental plaque disclosing agent and a radiopaque medium. It is commonly used in sweets and foods marketed to children, such as cake icing and cake-decorating gels. While commonly used in most countries of the world, erythrosine is rarely used in the United States (even though it has the FDA approval for use) due to its known hazards, with Allura Red AC being generally used instead.
FD&C Red No. 40	E129	Allura Red AC	Orange red	In the USA, Allura Red AC is approved by the FDA for use in cosmetics drugs & food, and also used in some tattoo inks. Can cause severe urticaria and dry skin rashes. Used in many products, such as soft drinks, children's medications, and candy floss. In Europe, Allura Red AC is not recommended for consumption by children. Banned in the UK, Denmark, Belgium, France, Switzerland, and Sweden.
FD&C Yellow No. 5	E102	Tartrazine	Lemon yellow	Commonly used colour all over the world, mainly for yellow, but can also be used with Brilliant Blue FCF, FD&C Blue 1, E133 or Green S (E142) to produce various green shades. Very widely used throughout the food processing industry, cosmetics, vitamins, antacids and medicinal prescription drugs.
FD&C Yellow No. 6	E110	Sunset Yellow FCF	Orange	It is a synthetic coal tar azo yellow dye Sunset Yellow is often used in conjunction with E123, Amaranth, in order to produce a brown colouring in both chocolates and caramel. Widely used in food processing and in medications. There have been repeated calls for the total withdrawal of Sunset Yellow from food use. EU & UK are working together to see that this happens by 2010.
Orange B				Orange B is a food dye from the azo dye group. It is approved by FDA for use only in hot dog & sausage casings or surfaces, only up to 150 ppm of the finished food weight. It usually comes as disodium salt
Citrus Red No2				Citrus Red 2, is an artificial dye. As a food dye, it is permitted by the FDA since 1956 only for use in the United States on the skin on some oranges. While the dye is a carcinogen, it does not penetrate the orange peel into the pulp. Citrus Red 2 is not water-soluble, but readily soluble in many organic solvents.
Information sourced from http://en.wikipedia.org				
A Consumer's Dictionary of Cosmetic Ingredients (ISBN 978-1-4000-5233-2) provides an excellent list of colours used in cosmetics				

Azo dyes

Azo compounds have vivid, high intensity colours, specifically reds, oranges and yellows. They are synthetic in origin and are more stable and colourfast than conventional vegetable based colourings.

Colour classifications

Colours are classified as either chemically organic or inorganic. This should not be confused with the other widely used definition "organic", which refers to growing or farming methods without the use of artificial pesticides, etc.

Organic colours (coal tar or anilines)

Organic colours were originally called coal tar or anilines because they were derived from coal sources. However, today almost all organic colours are synthetic and are available as water-soluble, oil-soluble or insoluble agents in all kinds of shades. Care must be taken when applying cosmetics that may contain coal tar derived colours, as these products are unsuitable for use on the lips or eyelids.

Inorganic colours

Inorganic, or "non-living" colours of insoluble metallic compounds which are derived from natural sources such as the earth (e.g. clay, carbon deposits, iron oxides etc).
Colours include browns, blacks, reds, ultramarines, chromium oxide green, mica, titanium dioxide, zinc oxide, etc).
Some of these are then subjected to high temperatures and some are bonded chemically with another elements, as in the case of titanium dioxide.

Confusingly, the natural colours also known as mineral pigments that are derived from the earth, are not technically considered "natural" because they are "inorganic" and have been treated or altered on a molecular level. Despite this, the aesthetic and beauty industry largely still term them natural even though this is not in principle, correct.

Inorganic colours do not posses the same kinds of health risks as organic colours; however, inorganic colours have a more limited colour range and are insoluble in water which has historically limited their range of applications. Intelligent encapsulation and other modern formulatory techniques have changed this.

Natural colours

Natural colours are derived or come directly from plant or animal sources, such as:
seeds (annatto); roots (turmeric); carbohydrates (caramel) leaves and stems (henna);
vegetables (such as red cabbage, beetroot juices, and carrot oil extract); fruits (grape juice); algae (ßeta carotene); insects (carmine).

Formulation review

Let us return to our sample formulation (below) to review the fragrances and colour additives used. Almost 24% of the individual ingredients in this formulation perform a fragrance or masking role. Our colour additive is playing the role of an opacifier. (Opaque or translucent in appearance) This type of opacity is often employed to convey the perception of purity. (Without additives)

1. Why do you think is it necessary to incorporate so many different fragrances in to the formulation?

2. How many of these individual fragrances are also found in fragrance mixes 1 or 2?

3. Which of these fragrances would accelerate post-inflammatory pigmentation?

4. How many may potentially have a negative effect on the skin?

Ingredients: Aqua, Glycerine, Niacinamide, Cetyl alcohol, Propylene glycol, Petrolatum, Cyclopentasiloxane, Isopropyl palmitate, Panthenol, Tocopherol acetate, Tocopherol, Camellia sinensis, Ceramide 3, Stearyl alcohol, Myristyl alcohol, Propylene glycol stearate, Titanium dioxide, Palmitic acid, Stearic acid, Dimethicone, Carbomer, Steareth-21, Steareth-2, Disodium EDTA, Sodium hydroxide, Aluminim hydroxide, Phenoxyethanol, Imidazolidinyl urea, Methylparaben, Propylparaben, Benzyl alcohol, Parfum, Hexyl cinnamal, Linalool, Hydroxyisohexyl 3-cyclohexene carboxaldehyde, Butylphenol methylpropional, Alpha-isomethyl ionone, Hydroxycitronellal, Geraniol, Citronellol, Limonene.

Compatability check list

	Fragrance	Fragrance fixing	Fragrance mix 1	Fragrance mix 2	Synthetic	Colour additive	Mandatory listing	Biomimetic	Occlusive	Antioxidant	Vitamin replacing	Restorative	Hydrating	Repair	Compromised skin
Aluminim hydroxide						✓									
Parfum	✓		✓			✓									
Benzyl alcohol		✓													
Hexyl cinnamal	✓			✓		✓									
Linalool	✓			✓		✓									
Hydroxyisohexyl 3-cyclohexene carboxaldehyde	✓		✓			✓									
Butylphenol methylpropional	✓			✓		✓									
Alpha-isomethyl ionone	✓			✓		✓									
Hydroxycitronellal	✓	✓				✓									
Geraniol	✓	✓				✓									
Citronellol	✓	✓				✓									
Limonene	✓					✓									

Ingredient specifications   Desirable criteria

Essential oils, botanicals & organics

There are literally hundreds of extracts and oils from plants that possess specific properties that are used in cosmetic formulations. The extracts and oils are derived from plants by the action of a variety of both ancient and modern techniques.

Botanical extracts and oils can contain a variety of actives including glycosides, polysaccharides, amino acids, enzymes and vitamins. The properties of most botanicals are positive. However it should be noted that there could be adverse side effects of some botanical extracts and oils that outweigh the benefits. Phototoxic reactions or post-inflammatory pigmentation may be caused by some botanicals under certain conditions.

What I'm trying to say here is that "natural" does not mean harmless, as many of your clients believe.

Botanicals are highly useful by the formulator because they offer a wide range of cosmetic ingredients; such as lipids (butters, oils, waxes, unsaponifiables), essential oils, tars, gums, mucilages, dyes, extracts etc.

The compound used for the preparation of plant extracts may be derived from the whole crude plant or some anatomical part; flower, leaf, fruit, bark, root or rhizome. Each extract contains dozens of chemicals in percentages that vary from season, zone, general weather, age of plant, harvest and storage. The range of actives may be classified into different chemical categories: acids, polyphenols, (tannins, flavonoids), terpenes, saponins, alkaloids, glycosides, amino acids, enzymes, metallic ions, alcohols, esters, carbohydrates, and phenols.

In order to have a functional topical action, the concentration of phyto-plant extracts differs according to the specific type of extract.

Without repeating too much of the information about the benefits of the" plant world" that is available to the clinician today, I have listed a few of the most common botanicals, essential oils and extracts and some of the essential oil carriers and emollients listed in groups according to some of their properties.

Essential oil extraction techniques

- Solvent
- Pressing
- CO2
- Forasols/Phytols

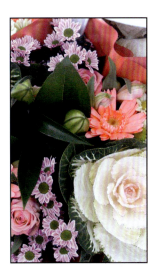

Healing - antiseptic and anti-microbial				
Thyme	Rosemary	Organum	Cumin	Sweet orange
Neroli	Lemon grass	Birch	Violet	Lavender
Melissa balm	Rose	Clove	Ylang ylang	Eucalyptus
Juniper	Peppermint	Sweet fennel	Rose geranium	Garlic
Meadowsweet	Lemon	Chinese anise	Cajeput	Orris
Sassafras	Cinnamon	Heliotrope	Wild thyme	Fir, Pine
Anise	Parsley	Mustard	Chinese cinnamon	Curry leaf

Dry skin extracts / oils				
St Johns wort	Elderflower	Aloe vera	Coltsfoot	Mallow
Quince	Acacia	Comfrey	Carrot	Orchid
Honey	Cornflower	Blackberry	Agrimony	Bearberry
Shinleaf	Clary sage	Honeysuckle	Strawberry	Roman
Chamomile	Kukui nut	Camellia	Evening primrose	Pomegranate

Oily skin - vasoconstricting and astringent				
Birch	Gentian	Witch hazel	Horsetail	Chamomile
Rosemary	Thyme	Great burdock	Hawthorn	Iceland moss
Peruvian bark	Cypress	Elderflower	Geranium	Yarrow
Calendula	Lovage	Sandalwood	Lemon	Salvia
Algae	Stinging nettle	Lemongrass	Lime	
Essential oil carriers – emollients				
Almond	Apricot	Avocado	Castor	Jojoba
Sunflower	Olive	Peach	Safflower	Sesame
Macadamia	Calendula	Barley	Caraway	Hazel
Flax seed				

Essential oils

Until recent times almost all terminology describing essential oils and their properties originate from the field of perfumery. The methodology of working with fragrant emollient esters such as essential oils became a profession in it's own right during the 1920's: The profession of Aromatherapy was born. Along with this came much of the same secrecy that had become part of the fragrance industry, with different distillation techniques and blends.

Today, the specialised knowledge about the therapeutic benefits of essential oils can be learned at reputable training institutes globally.

The UK still leads the world in setting standards and practice protocols, however this has not been enough to protect the public from the misuse of essential oils, nor has it prevented the flagrant adulteration of oils by some suppliers.

Genuine and authentic

If you are seeking the ultimate in superior quality essential oils, look for the classification "genuine and authentic". Essentially this designation should mean that they are pure, natural and complete crude oils which have not been re-distilled.

Moreover, they will have been distilled at a reduced pressure and heated as slowly and cautiously as possible to ensure maximum authenticity. Extraction in this way takes much longer and yields less oil per harvest, so this will obviously make the end product more expensive. The totally different quality of oil however, is well worth the price.

Adulteration of oils

Dilution or "extending" of essential oils is standard practice in many companies in order to make them cost efficient, however purists consider this to be adulteration. The extending is done with the introduction of a carrier oil, e.g. almond oil or the introduction of another "compatible" essential oil. Common "extending" include rose oil with geranium, and lavender oil with lavendin, with some companies still promoting the resultant blends as "pure" rose or lavender oil.

This kind of adulteration is very difficult to detect and often does not even show on a gas chromatogram as it is still basically an essential oil.

Another recent development is the use of emulsifiers (such as propylene glycol) to render the oils water-soluble. This is another form of extending, and allows the essential oil usable in vaporisers such as the Lucas Championnière.

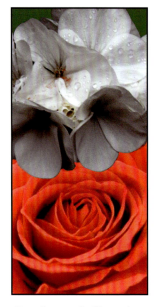

Extending rose oil with geranium, and lavender oil with lavendin is common practice.

Assessing oils containing carrier oils:

Here are some simple tests to help you detect extended oils.
Pure essential oils are highly volatile substances and are not greasy to touch. If you rub a little oil between your fingers and it leaves an oily film, this is an indication that it contains an extender. Another way to detect this type of extended oil is to place a drop of essential oil on a white sheet of paper. If it completely evaporates without the presence of a residue it should be a pure oil, however if it has been extended, it will leave an oily stain even after it dries.

Essential oils containing alcohol:

If an essential oil has been extended by the use of ethyl alcohol, you will only be able to identify it by detecting the characteristic odour of alcohol in the product.

Essential oils with emulsifiers:

To test an essential oil containing an emulsifier or surfactant, place a drop of essential oil in water. If it is pure, it will float to the top. If it contains a surfactant, it will dissolve in the water.
You must remember that pure essential oils are not miscible in water.

Labelling can be deceptive

Oils with the designation "pure, natural and complete: indicate that there are no other oils added (essential or carrier oils) and therefore making them pure. They do not contain synthetic materials, making them natural. They also have not undergone any de-colourising or de-terpensisation and are therefore complete. In other words they have not been tampered with or manipulated in any way. However they may, or may not be re-distilled.
There are several methods for ascertaining whether or not essential oils are genuine i.e. that they are truly volatile essential oils extracted from fresh plants. Some of these methods make use of the physical senses. The ability to detect the subtle differences through smell can be achieved by comparisons with samples of genuine oils of the same type.

Labelling some products as "aroma oils", "fragrance" or "perfumed" oils often means a poor quality product (Usually partially synthetic) that is blended for use in a diffuser to scent a room but not for any "contact" purpose such as to inhale, bathe in, or for use as body care.
Low quality essential oils have become part of daily lives; oil diffusers used to freshen rooms come in many forms from electric plug-ins, special quick melting oil-based candles or essential oil burners that are packaged with a small bottle of essential oil. The concern that comes from using low-grade blends or synthetic oils is that they have been adulterated with synthetically produced aromatic chemicals and these are released into the air along with the "so called essential oil".

Aromatherapy brings images being of safe and natural. However, true aromatherapy is not "safe" as there is a element of risk because of the influence the emollient esters can impart on the endocrine and nervous systems. Consequently, the use of full strength essential oils should never be practised by anyone who is not fully qualified. There are specific contrainications of various types of oils to health conditions (such as pregnancy) just as there are to medications.
Further, the sale of essential oils in department stores, on the internet and at pharmacies is of great concern, and many cases of misuse, over use, and post inflammatory pigmentation have resulted.
This will not get any better, and in fact will only get worse until it is recognised that essential oils and aromatherapy are methodologies that require long hours of study and should be practised only by individuals who have studied and fully understand the consequences of misuse.

Organic & natural

There will always be polarised discussion on the criteria of organic and natural ingredients in skin care products. Much of the traction that some marketers of "organic" and "natural" products obtain in the market comes from either statements or claims made on labels and promotional materials. These terms should not be confused with the same terms when used in reference to organic and natural foods; there is a big difference.

There are in excess of twenty different standards for "natural" cosmetics globally. The generally accepted criteria is that "natural" cosmetics contain 50% ingredients from a natural source, whilst "natural and organic" cosmetics contain a higher 95%.
Even this specification can be misleading when you consider that many so called "undesirable" substances (such as petroleum) are technically and chemically of "natural" origin.

For "certified organic" formulations, a maximum of 5% synthetic ingredients and a mere 5% and 10% minimum of certified organic ingredients is accepted, although in many parts of the world, any manufacturer can label a product as natural and organic, as there are very few regulating bodies, either government or private, that monitors or polices these label claims.
An example is a cosmetic product that has over 90% inorganic material and just 10% of an organic herb that could still state "organic" and "natural" on the label.

In cosmetic marketing, the terms "natural", "organic", "certified organic" and more commonly "??? free" implies that the formulation may be chemically different than other formulas with the same "non organic" or "synthetic" substances in them.
The reality of course is that molecules of the same chemical, be it from different origins are still the same molecular structure with the same properties, and there is no information available at this time that suggests substances that are from "organic" sources to be any different or safer than other chemicals with the same INCI (International Nomenclature of Cosmetic Ingredients) designation.
The exception is organic foods that have a distinct difference to commercially grown or produced substances.

Organic

The term "organic" when used in reference to cosmetics generally refers to a material that is produced without the use of preservatives, pesticides, chemical fertilisers, antibiotics or genetic enhancement. This is quite different from organic materials that are synthetically derived, and can cause confusion when trying to qualify the term "organic".
Consequently, from a marketing perspective, the word "organic" has become the new buzzword and superseded "natural" which can also be misrepresented to suit a marketing agenda.

There are however **genuine** organic ingredients available to formulators, and indeed **genuine** organic products on the market. The processes that are followed to produce organically certified ingredients are complex and controlled, with independent certifying bodies operating according to strict international standards. The entire process of product development is rigorously monitored beginning with the seed and how it is:

- Grown
- Harvested
- Stored
- Transported
- Processed

Providing each stage is completed according to international standards, then the finished product will display the certified organic logo from the relevant certifying body.
At times, there will be "hybrid" approaches to organic products; where the first crucial steps in

Organic Skin Care

The term "organic" refers to the type of chemistry used to describe the method of manufacture or physical description of the materials.

Essentially, organic chemistry is the science dealing with the element carbon and its compounds, and this should not be confused with the term "organic" that is used by the United States Department of Agriculture to describe the process or method by which some products or ingredients are grown or produced.

the organic process is respected, but the latter stages (such as final product processing) where conventional methods are employed.

Labelling deception

It is not uncommon for some cosmetic companies (both "natural" and conventional) to be "legally deceitful" (in accordance with US labelling regulations at least!) when formulating to achieve a particular labelling claim.

This occurs mostly where a product contains ingredients that are associated with beneficial properties without actually containing sufficient quantities of the ingredient to have any quantifiable effect.

This is achieved by the use of compounds that are designed specifically to help a formulation meet a labelling claim. A good example of this is vitamins, where the use of a compound containing less than .03% each of the three popular vitamins A, C & E is used in a cosmetic product to reach the threshold where the vitamin names can be legitimately listed on the label. (This compound would make up the minimum 1% of the total formulation)

The deception for the consumer is that while the formulation can be advertised as containing the beneficial vitamins, no mention of the minimum beneficial dose is made. In this scenario, the main purpose of the vitamin compound is to achieve the label claim, not to provide beneficial properties.

Green chemistry

Cosmetic chemists whose principles are to genuinely and realistically follow the "natural" and "organic" path subscribe to the principles of " green chemistry". This initiative offers the personal care industry an exciting opportunity to build brands on ethical principles while meeting compliances of safety, sustainability, and environmental concerns. Some of the twelve principles of green chemistry include:

- The design of chemical products to be fully effective, yet have little or no toxicity.
- Design syntheses to use and generate substances with little or no toxicity to humans and the environment.
- The use of catalysts, not stoichiometric reagents: catalysts are used in small amounts and can carry out a single reaction many times.
- Avoid chemical derivatives: avoid using blocking or protecting groups or any temporary modifications if possible. Derivatives use additional reagents and generate waste.
- Design syntheses so that the final product contains the maximum proportion of the starting materials.
- Avoid using solvents, separation agents, or other auxiliary chemicals.
- Design chemical products to break down to innocuous substances after use so that they do not accumulate in the environment.
- Include in-process real-time monitoring and control during syntheses to minimise or eliminate the formation of by-products, waste and pollution.

If you are considering embracing the green and natural philosophy in skin care products, there are many things to consider than just believing the label statements. I recommend you conduct due diligence on a proposed supplier with regard to the methods of manufacture, and bona fide material sources. Not all natural and organic product suppliers follow the core philosophy of natural and organic as scrupulously and conscientiously as perhaps they should.

"Green" Skin Care

The road leading to pure, natural & organic cosmetics is fraught with technical hurdles.

Formulation issues including performance, stability, safety, cost, and quality of raw material supply will always be the challenge when replacing synthetic chemicals with natural & organic alternatives.

Vitamins as actives

Vitamins are nutrients that are essential to life. By and large, vitamins function as co-enzymes, and enzymes are catalysts or activators in the chemical reactions that are continually taking place in our bodies. Vitamins are a fundamental part of these enzymes, bound up in proteins and minerals in a synergy and balance we need to survive.

These elements are now in cosmetic formulations and being presented in such a way that product composition links to skin structure and function, offering a corrective pathway based on biological fact, and not marketing hype.

Understanding the synergy of how one vitamin works with another, and that any loss of "the skin vitamin group" will reflect in the skin's health and appearance is valuable knowledge. The vitamin group consists of vitamins A, C, E, and B, and are supported by other vital skin nutrients such as the omega family and amino acids.

Why you don't see the word "vitamin" on the label

When looking at a label of any skin care cosmetic, you will not find the word "vitamin" on the label, and this is because international cosmetic labelling prohibits the use of the word "vitamin" in the ingredient list. An example is vitamin A, which will be most likely be listed as retinyl palmitate, or retinol.

Up until the mid 90's it was extremely difficult to stabilise and maintain the active action of a vitamin in a cosmetic formulation, and so very few formulations utilised vitamins. With the progress made with new formulatory techniques, liposomes and similar penetrating enhancing carriers, vitamins such as ascorbic acid (vitamin C) that oxidised easily are now stable and longer lasting in a cream. The use of vitamins has grown over the last decade to the point where we could not imagine treating skin or stocking a skin treatment line without a vitamin component.

The skin vitamin group: A,C & E

In this chapter, vitamins will be covered in a formulators manner and later in this book, many will be mentioned again in relation to a specific skin condition. Many vitamins have an emollient and humectant ability; and this makes them very useful from a formulator's point of view because the vitamin can be employed to perform multiple functions. These include being used as emulsifiers, emollients, humectants, antioxidants and of course, as actives. Vitamins also fit the "natural" and "green" image that so many consumers want.

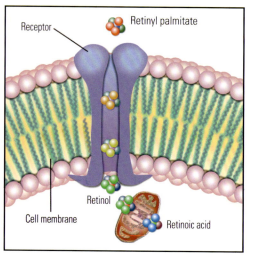

Receptor
Retinyl palmitate
Cell membrane
Retinol
Retinoic acid

Vitamin A

The ßeta-carotene pathway to retinoic acid

To begin this section on vitamins, we will begin with vitamin A. To truly understand vitamin A, it is important to understand carotenoids first, and the role they play in both skin and cosmetic formulations.

Carotenoids are a group of fat-soluble pigments widely distributed in plants and animals that act as precursors to vitamin A. These include lycopene, lutein, zeaxanthin and astaxanthin, and the widely studied and recognised ßeta-carotene.

The ßeta-carotene found in food is converted into vitamin A by absorption from the small intestine to the lymphatic system and transported and stored in the liver as retinyl palmitate until required.

It is delivered to the cells of the skin by conversion into retinol and attached to proteins in the bloodstream. Upon arrival in the extracellular spaces of the dermis/epidermis, it reverts to retinyl palmitate so it can enter the cell via special retinyl palmitate receptors. As it moves through the cell membrane it is further converted to retinol and finally to retinoic acid by the mitochondria.

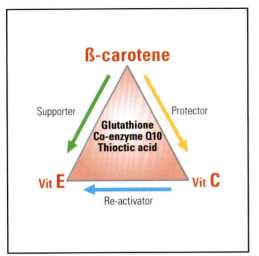

The vitamin group. Each interacts or plays a supporting role with another. Associated antioxidants are in the centre.

ßeta-carotene: pro vitamin A

ßeta-carotene is a precursor of vitamin A that belongs to the carotenoid group and is sometimes marketed as pro-vitamin A. As an antioxidant, ßeta-carotene is very stable, with one molecule able to counteract a vast number of free radicals, reducing sun damage and preventing lipid peroxidation. ßeta-carotene works in synergy with vitamin E and vitamin C, and is an important part of the antioxidant triangle (the vitamin group) of the epidermis.

Like vitamin E, ßeta-carotene is primarily used as an antioxidant or will be seen accompanying other antioxidants, such as vitamin C.

Recent nutritional research is showing that ßeta-carotene works in synergy with lycopene for optimal effect on cells and systems of the skin; this is why so many cosmetic chemistry formulators are now putting these two exciting carotenoids together to reduce lipid peroxidation.

Do not consider ßeta-carotene to be a "less than" effective ingredient in a cosmetic formulation. Carotenoids, such as ßeta-carotene, are natural antioxidant precursors of vitamin A.

In addition to it's role in vitamin A synthesis, ßeta-carotene has inherent photo-protective properties, and amalgamates well with both physical and chemical sun protection chemicals. Its ability to reduce UV-induced erythema will make ßeta-carotene a key player in the prevention and treatment of photo ageing and as a useful addition in after-sun products.

Vitamin A esters

The vitamin A that is found in large quantities in the extracellular space is the ester retinyl palmitate, which accounts for around 80% of the total vitamin A found in the skin.

The skins cells convert retinyl palmitate in to retinoic acid to sustain the DNA and cellular structures. This conversion occurs via a complex enzymic process shown in the simplified diagram at left. Consequently, the ester form of vitamin A plays a pivotal role in metabolism even though it is not used directly by the cells until conversion.

Because of the skin's ability to use this form of vitamin A, it is this form that is primarily found in topical application formulas.

Retinyl palmitate

The two forms of vitamin A frequently used in cosmetics are retinyl palmitate and retinyl acetate, with these esters proving less irritating to the skin while providing the same benefits and results as the more "aggressive" prescriptive versions of vitamin A such as tretinoin.

The natural ability to store vitamin A in the skin determines the level of retinoic acid that is found in the cells. Therefore, applying retinyl palmitate and other vitamin A esters such as ßeta carotene to the skin is an easy way to increase the amount of retinoic acid in the cells and to increase vitamin A receptors.

The ezymic process that converts ßeta carotene to the retinoic acid used by the cells

Studies show that up to 44% of the absorbed retinyl palmitate was hydrolysed into retinol, indicating that the topical use of retinyl palmitate results in significant delivery of retinol into the skin cell, and ultimately better skin health.

Retinyl palmitate has also been shown to exhibit a sun protection factor of 20, preventing sunburn, erythema and the formation of ROS (reactive oxygen species) radicals.

Retinol

Retinol is one of the most usable forms of vitamin A. (The alcohol form) In the body, the retinol form of vitamin A is an important "phase" because it is in the transitional form that it takes to travel from the liver to the dermis attached to proteins in the bloodstream.

It is this alcohol form of vitamin A that is regarded by many as the "true vitamin A" or "the complete molecule of vitamin A".

It is this belief that has encouraged the use of synthetic forms of retinol in skin care formulations, and despite being considered a "true" form of vitamin A, is not without its limitations, the most relevant being a short shelf life.

Retinol absorbs quickly into the skin from surface application, however hydrolyses to the retinyl palmitate form in the extracellular space to enter the cell via special receptors.

Retinoic acid

Retinoic acid is the acid form of vitamin A and has gained both great popularity and also notoriety. Despite chemically being the form of vitamin A directly used by the cells, it is the most irritating form, and usually procured only on prescription from a physician. Typical examples are Tretinoin or Renova. The side effects of topically applied retinoic acid can include redness, irritation, and flaking, and while impressive results have been achieved, client compliance is usually low with expectations not always met.

Vitamin A esters in the skin undergo a number of transitional stages before being finally used by the cells, with the conversion of retinol back to retinyl palmitate in the extracellular spaces an example. The biological and metabolic functions that regulate the use of vitamin A by the cells indicate that "rushing" the process will not always provide the best results.

Consequently, for optimal results with vitamin A esters and derivatives, acclimatising the keratinocytes and fibroblast cells by increasing vitamin A receptors, is the key to success. This will reduce the retinoid action and provide better client comfort.

Vitamin B

Vitamin B's are the new C's

In recent years, vitamin B has gained a great deal of attention from cosmetic chemists and is now being used extensively in all aspects of a cosmetic formulation from emollient properties through to anti-inflammatory agents. It has been commented that they are now enjoying the popularity that vitamin C once commanded.

The vitamin B group consists of over twelve individual vitamins, however there are eight that are commonly utilised in cosmetic and skin care formulations, more recently with the B7 and B9 groups.

- Vitamin B1 thiamine: used in shampoos and conditioners to help make hair shiny.
- Vitamin B2 riboflavin: principally used as a catalyst (chemical reaction accelerator).
- Vitamin B3 niacinamide: melanogenesis inhibitor (inhibits melanosome transfer).
- Vitamin B5 panthenol: penetrating moisturiser, anti-inflammatory agent.
- Vitamin B6 pyridoxine: hair care products (labelled as pyridoxine hydrochloride).
- Vitamin B6 pyridoxine tripalmitate: stable oil soluble form of B6 with emollient properties.
- Vitamin B7 biotin: recent addition to facial creams, hair and nail care products.
- Vitamin B9 folic acid (folocin):   recent addition to facial creams, hair and nail care products.

Vitamin B3

Most commonly known as niacin, niacinamide and nicotinic acid, this water soluble vitamin shows a stabilising effect on epidermal barrier function and a reduction in TEWL. As a by-product of increasing cell energy and assisting DNA repair, there is a increase in protein synthesis and a stimulating effect on ceramide synthesis. This leads to enhanced epidermal cell turnover and healthier appreaing skin.
Niacinamide is also an effective melanogenesis inhibiting compound that works by preventing melanosome transfer from melanocytes to keratinocytes.

Vitamin B5

This is the most frequently used form of vitamin B in cosmetic formulations because of its many properties. After application, B5 panthenol converts to pantothenic acid (B complex vitamin) promoting normal keratinisation and wound healing. It is this property that makes it useful for the relief of sunburn, itching, mild eczema and dermatitis.

The vitamin B complex also aids in the water retention powers of the skin due to its humectant properties, and is soluble in both water and alcohol. The pro-vitamin and water-soluble aspects of panthenol combine to yield a non-irritant, non-sensitising, moisturising and conditioning feel, and it is found as the "wonder ingredient" in some well known department store and supermarket brands.
In this guise it is known as calcium d-Pantothenate, (natural pro-vitamin B5) or Pro-calcium™.

Vitamin C: ascorbic acid

Vitamin C has been in the spotlight for nearly two decades, and over that time has evolved from being a very difficult ingredient to employ into a cosmetic formulation, to one that is found in many anti-ageing creams in the skin treatment industry today.
This place in the industry did not come about without a lot of discussion, comparisons, and what at the time, seemed like industrial espionage.

Ascorbic acid is utilised by cells as an antioxidant, and in a more complicated way, is used to assist the fibroblast in making collagen. We discuss this process in more depth in chapter two.

Vitamin C in cosmetic formulations takes one of five major forms, each with differing properties, but all are used for the single purpose of delivering ascorbic acid to the skin cells. Vitamin C's are used in both water and lipid soluble forms and when applied topically, are far more efficient than massive doses of oral supplements.
As vitamin C has a very short "active" period and oxidised easily, it needs to be replenished daily both topically and nutritionally.

Among the properties of vitamin C is the protection of vitamin A against oxidation and the conversion of inactivated vitamin E back into its active antioxidant form.

One of the most interesting properties is its ability to inhibit melanin formation. By blocking the action of the enzyme tyrosinase, it inhibits all future steps of melanogenesis. It is also now well known that the skin gets considerably less damage if significant amounts of vitamin C are applied topically before and after sun exposure.

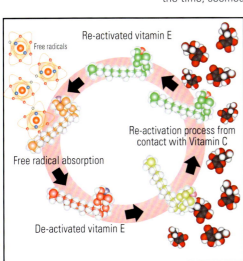

Re-activated vitamin E

Free radicals

Re-activation process from contact with Vitamin C

Free radical absorption

De-activated vitamin E

The re-activation or protection of vitamin E
as an active ant-oxidant by vitamin C

Types of Vitamin C

L-ascorbic acid, ascorbic acid:

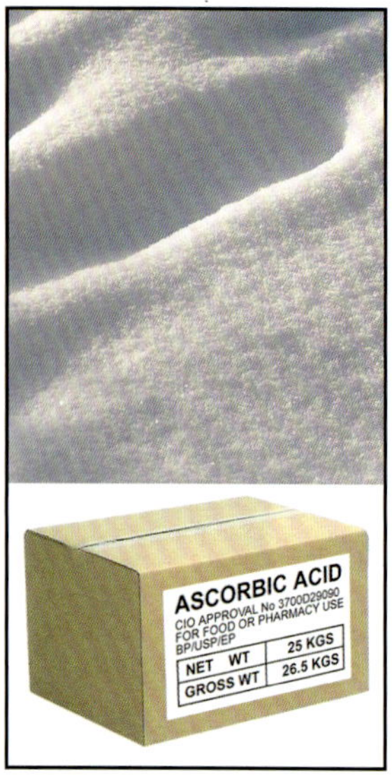

The most common form of topical vitamin C is L-ascorbic acid, which is a chiral molecule (refer section at the end of vitamins). In nature, vitamin C only exists in the L- configuration of chirallity, with the synthetic variety of ascorbic acid used in skin care formulations produced with both L- and D- molecular structures.

Pure forms of L- ascorbic acid (with just the L- molecule) are created by specialised processing of ascorbic acid that excludes the D- molecule. It is only these "purified" versions of the ascorbic acid that can be considered real or "natural" L-ascorbic acid.

It is not uncommon for manufacturers to claim to be using L-ascorbic acid, when in reality they are using unpurified ascorbic acid with both L- and D- molecular structures.

Traditional synthesis of ascorbic acid is through a process which requires bioconversion of sorbitol followed by a seven-step chemical process. However newly developed fermentation technology is currently used to reduce production costs.

Ascorbic acid solutions, as its name implies, has an acidic pH. Under natural conditions the pH can easily be 2 or lower, depending on the concentration. In greater saturation, the resultant lower pH renders the solution more stable, however this is at the expense of being more of an irritant to the skin, and the main reason why ascorbic acid is not the first choice for compromised skins.

Ascorbyl palmitate (ascorbyl di palmitate)

Ascorbyl palmitate is the most widely used oil-soluble (lipophilic) derivative of vitamin C in skin care products, and is formed from ascorbic acid and palmitic acid creating an oil-soluble, ester form of the vitamin.

It is also known as vitamin C palmitate, L-ascorbyl-6-palmitate and 3-oxo-L-gulofuranolactone 6-palmitate. Being oil soluble, it is readily attracted to the oil phases of the skin where it acts as an antioxidant to protect the cell membranes.

Ascorbyl palmitate works in synergy with vitamin E in the prevention of lipid peroxidation, and also well in sun protection formulations by improving the skin's resistance to the damaging effects of the sun. The use of ascorbyl palmitate in anti-ageing medicine was pioneered by the two times Nobel Laureate Dr. Linus Pauling, whose research and subsequent clinical studies showed that ascorbyl palmitate, when used in combination with vitamin C and amino acids, lysine and proline, is able to strengthen the vascular wall and supporting connective tissue.

Aminopropyl ascorbyl phosphate

A new derivative with the same benefits as ascorbic acid, but with reported longer shelf life, low acidity and stability. This form of vitamin C will have easy access in to a cell via the ion receptors for phosphate. Similarly to MAP, this form of vitamin C will be suitable for compromised, high risk skins and likely to be seen in future skin lightening and anti-ageing products.

Ascorbyl glucoside

Ascorbyl glucoside has a structure in which the C2-hydroxyl group of ascorbic acid is masked with glucose. After absorption into the skin, the ascorbyl glucoside is reduced into ascorbic acid and glucose by the enzyme, alpha-glucosidase. The resulting ascorbic acid component exhibits antioxidant activity, and acts as a co-enzyme for enzymes involved in collagen synthesis, (prolyl and lysyl hydroxylase) and inhibits the synthesis of melanin. It has also been used in conjunction with niacinamide (B3) with favourable results in skin lightening products.

The vitamin C used in cosmetic formulations is far different to that associated with fruit & vegetables, and quality varies considerably dependant on source.

Ascorbic acid limitations

One of the limiting factors in the use of ascobic acid in cosmetics and skin care is its relatively short shelf life.

This means that "fresh" product is required constantly, and stockpiling is a waste of time.

Despite claims of superior stabilisation by some manufactures, all ascorbic acid solutions will lose potency after around six months, even if strict temperature and dark storage conditions are met.

Be sure to check your "use by" dates during monthly stocktakes.

Magnesium ascorbyl phosphate (MAP)

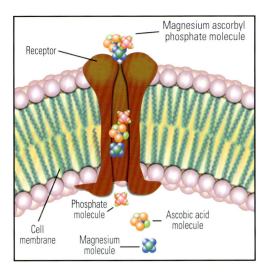

Magnesium ascorbyl phosphate molecule

Receptor

Phosphate molecule

Ascobic acid molecule

Cell membrane

Magnesium molecule

This is a water-soluble (hydrophilic) compound that is gaining increasing popularity with skin care formulators because of it's negligible skin irritation and stability. Magnesium ascorbyl phosphate is reported to exhibit the same potential as ascorbic acid to improve skin collagen synthesis, but is effective in significantly lower concentrations (less acidic).
This is because the combination of ascorbic acid and magnesium (or sodium) and phosphate "trick" the cells to uptake a higher dose than just ascorbic acid alone. Once inside the cells, the compound is converted to its individual elements and used within the cell.

Magnesium ascorbyl phosphate is considered a better choice than ascorbic acid for individuals with compromised, high risk skin and those wishing to avoid any of the associated exfoliating effects encountered with ascorbic acid.
Magnesium ascorbyl phosphate, as a raw material, is generally more expensive than ascorbic acid and therefore not always readily found in domestic retail (department store) products, but is becoming widely used in the professional skin care industry.

Ascorbyl tetraisopalmitate

Ascorbyl tetraisopalmitate (AKA tetrahexyldecyl ascorbate) is another lipid soluble (lipophilic) version of vitamin C and consequently extremely stable. The name tetraisopalmitate indicates that there are four molecules of palmitic acid attached to the ascorbic acid molecule.
Because the ascorbic acid is the "smaller" component of the compound, it is less acidic and less irritating, and the fat solubility allows it to pass more easily through the bilayers of the stratum corneum and reach the target cell walls. The oil solubility means that increased amounts of active vitamin C reach the cells.
Ascorbyl tetraisopalmitate works well in formulations in conjunction with vitamin A, and has an excellent shelf life.

Sodium ascorbyl phosphate

Sodium ascorbyl phosphate is a water soluble (Hydrophilic) derivative of ascorbic acid, which has improved stability arising from its chemical structure. In the skin, it is converted into free ascorbic acid by a similar enzymatic process that converts retinyl palmitate to retinoic acid.
Sodium ascorbyl phosphate is shown to be effective in scavenging oxidising agents, and has proven effective in treating acne scarring in Asian skins. It has been shown to work well with iontophoresis.

Other vitamin C derivatives

There are a number of other vitamin C derivatives used in formulations for their antioxidant properties, with ascorbyl stearate (an ester of ascorbic acid and stearic acid), erythorbic acid/isoascorbic acid (an isomer of ascorbic acid) and sodium erythorbate, (the sodium salt of erythorbic acid) the most common.

Isomers

Any of two or more substances that are composed of the same elements in the same proportions, but differ in properties because of differences in the arrangement of atoms.

Vitamin E

Vitamin E is a family of oil soluble (lipophilic) antioxidants that protect against lipid peroxidation. Two sub-groups of the vitamin are tocopherols and tocotrienols, and the name vitamin E is often the generic term used to describe both. In each group there are four natural variations designated as alpha, ßeta, gamma and delta. An example is the widely studied a-tocopherol (also known as alpha-tocopherol) .

True linking product composition to skin structure and function is seen with the action that vitamin E exhibits in cosmetic formulations as an antioxidant, emollient and active ingredient.
Vitamin E is an effective antioxidant, however in the role of protecting the skin, can only neutralise one free radical at a time. Other antioxidants such as vitamins C, A and alpha-lipoic acid are required to reactivate a-tochopherol back to its active form.

Tocopherol has traditionally been only soluble in alcohol, fats, and oils, and like vitamin A palmitate, it can be emulsified in aqueous solutions with emulsifiers such as polysorbitate 80. There is now a new form of vitamin E that is water soluble: Vitamin E TPNa INCI: Sodium tocopheryl phosphate. This new compound has all of the benefits of oil soluble vitamin E, with the expanded formulatory opportunities a water soluble version brings.
In cosmetic formulations vitamin E is commonly listed in the formulation under the name of tocopherol usually in companion with ascorbic acid. This is because of the synergistic nature of these two vitamins in both in skin and formulations. (See page 67)

Tocopherol group

Rather than tocopherol itself, esters of tocopherol are often used in cosmetic and personal care products. These esters include:

* Tocopheryl acetate: the acetic acid ester of tocopherol.
* Tocopheryl glucoside: emollient.
* Tocopheryl linoleate: the linoleic acid ester of tocopherol, has been shown to offer increased emollient and humectant properties when used in moisturisers.
* Tocopheryl linoleate/oleate: a mixture of linoleic and oleic acid esters of tocopherol
* Tocopheryl nicotinate: the nicotinic acid ester of tocopherol.
* Tocopheryl succinate: the succinic acid ester of tocopherol.
* Potassium ascorbyl tocopheryl phosphate: a salt of both vitamin E (tocopherol) and vitamin C. (Ascorbic acid) may also be used in cosmetic products.
* Tocopherol phosphate mixture: used as a delivery system due to amphillic properties.
* Sodium tocopheryl phosphate: water solubility will expand formulatory uses of vitamin E.

Tocotrienols

Despite being the least studied variety of vitamin E, some research suggests tocotrienols are more potent in their anti-oxidation effect than the common forms of tocopherol, due to significant differences in chemical structure. The unsaturated side-chain in tocotrienols helps them penetrate tissues with bilayers more efficiently, giving them greater potential for use in cosmetic products.

Tocopherols are generally present in common vegetable oils (i.e. soy, canola), while tocotrienols are concentrated in cereal grains. (ie. oat, barley, rye and rice bran) The highest levels are found in crude palm oil. Commercial tocotrienols and tocopherols are mainly obtained from natural sources, such as palm or rice bran oil.

Chirally correct?

The "chirally correct" status of compounds used in skin care formulations can be a subject of great debate. While the claims of superior effectiveness of chiral molecules has some scientific basis, some of the "chirally correct" ingredients in the formulations are not in reality what they seem.

So what is chirality? What is the relevance in skin care formulations?
The term chirality refers to the way a compounds molecular structure wraps around an axis.
The strings of molecules that make up the compound can either rotate around the axis in a left or right handed direction. These compounds are called "enantiomers" of each other, meaning they have the same number of each type of molecule but are configured in a slightly different way in space.

Put simply, these "chiral" compounds are not symmetrical, and are not super imposable with its mirror image. The human hand is the most widely used example of this: left and right hands that have a thumb, fingers in the same order, but are mirror images of each other and not the same. This is exemplified by trying to put a left-hand glove on a right hand. Same shape, but not the same fit. Chiral molecules have the same elements attached in the same order, but are mirror images and not the same. The example amino acid graphic (at lower left) shows this configuration.

In chemistry, the configuration of the molecules is identified by a R- or S- , however most chiral substances found in skin care are identified by the L- and D- naming convention where the left hand molecule is known as the "L-" (or levo) and the right hand is known as the "D-" (or dextro) molecule.

The "chiral" status

The regulations of COLIPA (European Trade Association representing the cosmetics industry) and soon, the CTFA (Cosmetics, Toiletries & Fragrance Association) prohibit the declaration of the chiral status of a molecule in formulation marketing.

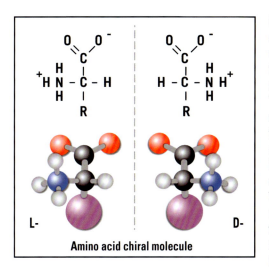

Amino acid chiral molecule

So what does it all mean? Chirality has implications for chemical synthesis of pharmaceuticals and other substances because some chirally configured materials will work more efficiently than others because the body has receptors that can only interact with molecules in a specific shape. (L- or D- form depending on which the receptors will more readily recognise.
The proteins in higher animals (including humans) are made from L-amino acids, coded for right handed helical DNA containing only D sugars. (This is why DNA twists as it does) Similarly, enzymes synthesised in the body are also "L-" configuration.
Most organisms (including plants) tend to synthesize more of the L-rotated compounds, and it is believed that L- configured molecules are more efficient. When a substance is chirally correct, this means that it contains only the molecules with the ability to interact more efficiently with the receptors at the target site in order to give the designed results (either the D or the L form). However the difference in effectiveness may only be small in some cases, as our biological systems recognise and use compounds with both chiralities.

Some marketers of skin care formulations have embraced the term chirally correct to help raise the profile of their formulations, they have however taken liberties with the facts surrounding chiral molecules to "embellish" the facts with pseudo science for their own needs.

An example of a spurious chiral molecule is L-retinol. You will never find a reference to it in a chemistry book because it is not a chemical reality. Retinoids belong to a different group of isomers to that of the chiral molecule L-ascorbic acid belongs to. Isomers have the same molecular formula, but different structural formulas. In fact, the term "L-retinol" is a trade-mark, and nothing more than a cunning marketing strategy.

Antioxidants

There are two severe levels of cellular damage that occur from the free radicals that aggravate many skin conditions; oxidative stress and lipid peroxidation. Before we embark on discussing antioxidants, a brief review of these two forms of cellular damage is appropriate to help put things into perspective.

We know that cells are normally able to defend themselves against ROS damage through the use of enzymes such as superoxide dismutases, catalases, glutathion peroxidases (extracellular) and peroxiredoxins.   It is the depletion of these intrinsic antioxidant resources that leads to lipid peroxidation and further cellular damage from which the cell may not recuperate, or have the resources to recover from.

What is oxidative stress?

Oxidative stress is the loss of both oil and water soluble antioxidants within the immediate environment around the protective membrane. Examples of these are vitamin E, thioctic acid (alpha lipoic acid), omega's 3 & 6, (in the form of essential fatty acids), vitamin A, (in the form of retinyl palmitate and beta carotene) and vitamin C.

Although vitamin E abounds in quantity, it is a very poor antioxidant and can only neutralise a small number of free radicals before becoming inactive. Vitamin E is reactivated by vitamin C and therefore without vitamin C, the cell has lost an important antioxidant (vit E) leaving it susceptible to oxidative stress. This then leads on to lipid peroxidation, which is a deterioration of the phospholipids that make up 45% of the cell membrane.

UVR in the form of sunburn is a common primary cause of oxidative stress as is ingestion of alcohol and cigarettes. All of these are sources of the highly reactive hydroxyl radicals.

The first changes that occurs in the skin after chronic or acute UV irradiation is the generation of reactive oxygen species, (ROS) leading to the peroxidation of unsaturated lipids (Including the loss of oil soluble antioxidants) in the cell membrane.

Lipid peroxidation can lead to mitochondria DNA damage (M/DNA)

Put simply, lipid peroxidation is a compounded and untreated intracellular form of oxidative stress that includes cell membrane phospholipids and the loss of oil soluble antioxidants. All cells can be influenced in a negative way, so much so that a vicious cycle begins, and over time, this will lead to more serious cellular damage such as mitochondria DNA damage of a cell. As an example, in the condition of pigmentation it will be the melanocyte and keratinocyte cell most affected.

The mitochondria is considered the "power house" of a cell, and this vital part of the cell interior is surrounded by a delicate cell membrane. This smaller cell membrane is attached to part of the outer cell membrane in places such as the endoplasmic reticulum. What this means is that if lipid peroxidation is left to compound and the outer cell membrane compromised, the interior of the cell is next to be affected.

Once affected, the mitochondria cell membrane may become permanently damaged, leaving cellular production and energy at risk, resulting in the cell's memory becoming compromised and very difficult to correct. As a result, the cell may mutate or undergo apoptosis (Cell death)

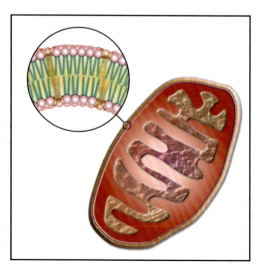

Around the outside and interior of the mitochondria is an important cell membrane that is susceptible to intracellular oxidative stress.

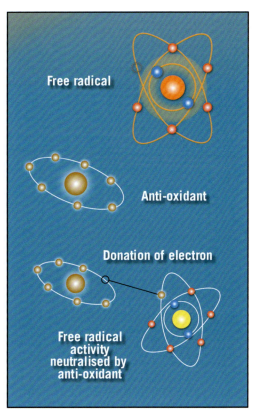

Free radical

Anti-oxidant

Donation of electron

Free radical
activity
neutralised by
anti-oxidant

Antioxidants are compounds that protect cells against the damaging effects of reactive oxygen species (ROS) such as singlet oxygen, superoxide, peroxyl radicals, hydroxyl radicals and peroxynitrite. An imbalance between antioxidants and reactive oxygen species results in oxidative stress, and consequent cellular damage.

Linking product composition to skin structure and function

The relative importance and interactions between different antioxidants is a complex area, with the various metabolites and enzyme systems having synergistic and interdependent effects on one another. The action of one antioxidant may depend on the proper function of other members of the antioxidant system, and the amount of protection provided by any one antioxidant therefore depends on its concentration, its reactivity towards the particular reactive oxygen species being considered, and the status of the antioxidants with which it interacts.

There are two main groups of antioxidants; (hydrophilic) water soluble or (hydrophobic) oil soluble, and in general, the following principles apply:

- Water-soluble antioxidants react with oxidants in the cell, (Intracellular) and outside the cell. (Extracellular)
- Lipid-soluble antioxidants protect cell membranes from lipid peroxidation and work in synergy with the water-soluble group.

Not all enzymes, proteins, vitamins and metabolites can be used as actives in cosmetic chemistry. However, what should be understood is what specific cells of various systems require to function efficiently. This knowledge will help choose an antioxidant most effective for a particular condition. An example is oxidative stress that causes lipid peroxidation and subsequent lipofuscin formation. (Glycation of cell membrane proteins and cellular waste)

It is difficult to find an element that exactly matches each one of the skins own antioxidants systems, however there will be an enzyme or vitamin that is a co-factor that may make a difference.
In this segment I am trying to avoid talking about these antioxidants as nutritional supplements and only wish to write of those that are known to be useful and proven in a topical format. Having already covered vitamins used successfully in cosmetic formulations in the previous pages, there will be limited repeat discussion in this segment.
The following sections discuss antioxidants that are similar or have an affinity to the intrinsic antioxidants that reside in the immediate environs of the cell membranes, and are being successfully used in cosmetic formulations.

Super oxide dismutase (SOD) as an intracellular antioxidant

Also known as super dismutase oxide, this is an enzyme that protects against oxidative stress, functioning as a prime scavenger of free radicals. It has the capability of preventing fats from changing into harmful lipid peroxide, making this enzyme important both inside the cells and cell membranes.
There are three forms of superoxide dismutase in our cells. SOD1 is located in the cytoplasm (cell interior), SOD2 in the mitochondria and SOD3 is extracellular. Each of these contain different elements in their reactive centres, with SOD1 and SOD3 containing copper and zinc, and SOD2 containing manganese.
Unfortunately this built-in defence system declines with age, and as part of any anti-ageing strategy, it would be greatly beneficial to include a formulation containing super dismutase oxide.

Coenzyme Q10, Ubiquinone (AKA Idebenone)

This oil-soluble vitamin-like substance is present in most skin cells, primarily in the mitochondria. It is a component of the electron transport chain and participates in aerobic cellular respiration, generating energy in the form of the coenzyme Adenosine-5'-triphosphate (ATP).

Idebenone is an analogue or synthetic equivalent coenzyme Q10 (Co Q10) and is more water-soluble than Co Q10. Its cellular distribution and antioxidant profile are also rather different too, and this renders idebenone superior to Co Q10 in neutralizing some types of free radicals and inferior in fighting other types; especially those that damage the cell membrane.
Idebenone may be listed on some product labels as hydroxydecyl ubiquinone and is showing to be very successful when used in sun protection formations. Research has seen reduction in the MMP enzyme collagenase (denatures collagen fibril) which is accelerated by exposure to UVA.

Thioctic acid (alpha lipoic acid)

Thioctic acid is an organic compound classed as a carboxylic acid. It is also known as A-lipoic acid, 5-(Dithiolan-3-yl) Valeric acid, as well as 1,2-Dithiolane-3-Pentanoic acids. But the most popular and recognised name is alpha lipoic acid.
Thioctic acid is a unique radical protector with high bioavailability for all cells because it is both oil and water-soluble, it can easily travel across cell membranes to fight free radicals both inside (intracellular) and outside (extracellular) the cell.

As thioctic acid works both inside the cell and at the membrane level, any free radicals that make it past the first line of protection are combated right inside the cell itself.
Thioctic acid is firstly a coenzyme in the metabolic process and is necessary for the conversion of glucose to energy (ATP) making it an important part of the mitochondria.
Thioctic acid works together with other antioxidants such as vitamins C, E and ßeta carotene, and as a "recycler" some vitamins. As an example, when vitamin E quenches lipid peroxidation, a vitamin E radical is formed, and that radical is reduced back to a re-activated vitamin E by the lipoic acid.
It also performs a similar task with vitamin C. A very special metabolite indeed!

Glutathione (amino acid)

Glutathione is an important intracellular antioxidant that protects against a variety of different radical species and is a compound classified as a tripeptide made of three amino acids: cysteine, glutamic acid and glycine.
Ascorbic acid and glutathione work well together as antioxidants in all areas around the cell membrane, both inside and out, and on the cell membrane itself. The role of the ascorbic acid is protecting the glutathione from oxidation. This is important to remember when linking product composition to skin structure & function.

The right choice of vitamin C as a protective companion to glutathione is important, as one that would be quickly absorbed and have an immediate effect on the cell membrane and intracellular structures would provide the most benefit.
As the cell membrane is a double layer of lipid molecules, it would be easy to see a lipid soluble form of vitamin C would be the most efficient.
Ascorbyl tetra-isopalmitate or ascorbyl palmitate would be the first to choices.

The ORAC scale: The antioxidant point of reference

ORAC stands for Oxygen Radical Absorbance Capacity, and is a test developed to measure the antioxidant speed and power of foods and supplements. The ORAC test is quickly becoming the accepted standard for comparing antioxidant capacity.
To date, essential oils have shown to have the highest ORAC ratings. A sample cross section of scores includes:

Clove oil:	1,078,700
Patchouli:	49,400
Vitamin E oil:	3,309
Blueberries:	2,400
Carrots:	210

Will the ORAC scale ever be used to score antioxidants in cosmetic formulations? Only time will tell..

Antioxidant nutrients

Selenium and zinc are commonly referred to as antioxidant nutrients, however these chemical elements have no antioxidant properties themselves. They are instead used for the activation of some antioxidants enzyme.

Ergothioneine

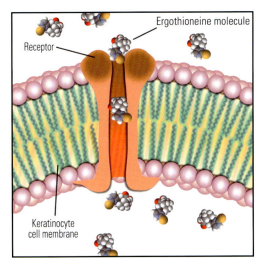

Ergothioneine molecule

Receptor

Keratinocyte
cell membrane

One of the "Generation Z" antioxidants, ergothioneine (EGT) is a naturally-occurring amino acid that derived from fungi (mushrooms) or animal tissue sources.

Researchers have found L-ergothioneine to be more efficient in inhibiting lipid peroxide formation than coenzyme Q10 or its synthetic analog idebenone.

It is reported to act significantly quicker and more efficiently in capturing ROS, and this may be because it is different than most antioxidants in that keratinocytes have receptors that allow it to penetrate the cell wall, while most other antioxidants perform their functions in the extracellular matrix.

Botanicals as antioxidants

Many if not most of the antioxidants that are used in the cosmetic industry come from botanical origins, and categorising the actions of botanical antioxidants is difficult because they are too many to mention. Most botanical antioxidants can be classified into one of three categories; flavonoids, carotenoids and polyphenols.

Flavonoids / Bioflavonoids

Flavonoids possess a polyphenolic structure that accounts for their antioxidant, UV protectant, and metal chelation abilities. Bioflavonoids work with other antioxidants to offer a system of protection. Numerous studies have shown their unique role in protecting vitamin C from oxidation in the body, thereby allowing the body to reap more benefits from vitamin C.

Silymarin as a flavonoid

This extract consists of 3 flavonoids derived from the fruit, seeds, and leaves of the milk thistle plant (Silybum marianum), which belongs to the aster family of plants, including daisies, thistles, and artichokes.

These flavonoids are used as antioxidants in a pre-emptive role to avoid cellular damage before it starts, rather than "mopping up" existing damage. It is used homeopathically to treat some disease, and is a strong antioxidant that prevents lipid peroxidation.

Polyphenols as antioxidants

Polyphenols compose the largest category of botanical antioxidants. The most widely used commercialised polyphenol antioxidants are:

- Epigallocatechin gallate (EGCG) (from green & white tea)
- Ferulic Acid
- Resveratrol
- Hypericin (St. John's wort)
- Chlorogenic acid (blueberry leaf)
- Caffeic acid
- Rosmarinic acid (rosemary)
- Ellagic acid (pomegranate fruit)
- Oleuropein (olive leaf)

Common Flavones

- Rutin & Quercetin
  (apples, blueberries)
- Hesperidin & Diosmin
  (lemons, oranges)

Common Xanthones

- Mangiferin
  (mango plant)

- Mangostin
  (bilberry plant)

Curcumin

Curcumin is a polyphenol antioxidant derived from the turmeric root. It is sometimes used in skin care products as a natural yellow colouring in products that claim to be free of artificial ingredients. Tetrahydrocurcumin, a hydrogenated form of curcumin, is off-white in colour and can be added to skin care products not only to function as a skin antioxidant, but also to prevent the lipids in the moisturiser from becoming rancid. The antioxidant effect of tetrahydrocurcumin is reported by some cosmetic chemists to be greater than vitamin E.

Resveratrol (INCI: 3,4',5-trihydroxystilbene)

Resveratrol is a polyphenol related to curcumin, and found in red grape skins, raspberries and blueberries. It is a antioxidant, anti-inflammatory and improves glycation.
In it's role as an antioxidant, it reduces damage to endothelial cells exposed to nitrite radicals and protects skin cells against damage caused by UV radiation. It also inhibits lipid peroxidation of low-density lipoproteins.
Like carnosine, it offers all of the benefits of anti-ageing and antioxidants, but mostly from a supplemental standpoint. Although potentially a good candidate for cosmetic formulations, it is however generally unstable in formulations due to it hydrolyzing and causing discoloration. Accordingly, it is generally only used in very small amounts unless it has been derivatized. (To alter it's chemical composition to a derivative)

Ferulic acid (INCI: 4-hydroxy-3-methoxycinnamic acid)

Also known as cinnamic acid, this is a antioxidant which neutralises the superoxide, nitric oxide, hydroxyl radicals and helps to prevent cell damage from UVR. Paradoxically, exposure to ultraviolet light actually increases ferulic acid's antioxidant potency. The chemical structure of ferulic acid is very similar to that of curcumin. With this profile, it should work well with sun protection products.
In Japan, the concentration of Ferulic acid is restricted in some cosmetics.

Xanthones as antioxidants

Xanthones exhibit strong antioxidant activity, and are thought to be more potent than both vitamin C and vitamin E. Often referred to as the "Super Antioxidants", Xanthones have been found to support and enhance the body's immune system. They are heat stable molecules and unlike proteins, won't denature or lose their structure when heated. This property should make them a useful addition to sun protection and other formulations exposed to radiant heat.

Carotenoids

In addition to ßeta-carotene, lutein, lycopene and astaxanthin, there are also the colourless carotenoids; phytoene and phytofluene from algae and tomato sources that are also UV protectants and antioxidants.

Common Carotenoids

- Astaxanthin
  (algae, tomatoes)

- Carotene
  (pumpkin, carrots)

- Lutein & Lycopene
  (tomatoes)

New antioxidants: Spin traps

Spin traps are compounds that as the name suggests, have the ability to stabilise or "trap" free radicals, and so reduce their cascade effect on other molecules.

The more technical term for the spin traps would be radical scavenger, as the compounds effectively grab the free radicals and pull them in to the spin trap mass.

Researchers studying spin traps discovered that the fundamental mechanism of "spin trap" activity is different from other anti-oxidants. In most conventional antioxidants, the compounds "destructively" act upon the free radicals by chemically reacting with them to convert the ROS (reactive oxygen species) into water.

Conversely, spin traps "constructively" deal with the ROS in a passive way by intercepting them before any damage is done. This is perhaps why some researchers have dubbed the spin traps as the "intelligent" antioxidant, as they are the only antioxidants that differentiate between good oxygen molecules and injurious ones (ROS).

Spin traps can complement other skin anti-ageing treatments. It is understood that both topical vitamin C and alpha-hydroxy acids, such as glycolic and lactic acid, generate hydroxyl free radicals, and the inclusion of spin traps in to the formulations may potentially reduce any negative effects. The spin trap PBN (Phenyl-butyl-nitrone) has shown to scavenge the free radicals produced by alpha-hydroxy-acids, and the spin trap TEMPO trap free radicals produced by vitamin C.

Technically, true spin traps are "nitrone" or a "nitroso" compounds such as PBN or "Phenyl-butyl-nitrone", so when looking at formulations that claim to contain spin trap technology, at least one of these nitrone and nitroso spin trap compounds should be present:

- N-tert-butyl-alpha-phenylnitrone (PBN)
- 3,5-dibromo-4-nitrosobenzenesulfonic acid
- 2-methyl-2-nitrosopropane
- alpha.-(4-pyridyl-1-oxide)-N-t-butylnitrone
- 2,4,6-tri-t-butylnitrosobenzene

- 2,2,6,6-Tetramethylpiperidine-N-Oxyl (TEMPO)
- 5,5-dimethyl-1-pyrroline N-oxide
- Nitrosodisulfonic acid
- 3,3,5,5-tetramethylpyrroline N-oxide

Despite spin traps demonstrating affects on cellular oxidation states and oxidative sensitive enzyme systems, it is still perhaps too early (at the time of writing this book) to conclusively prove that they have a markedly superior effect as an anti-ageing agent than the antioxidants currently in use.

Spin trap superiority?

It is theorised that an over abundance of conventional antioxidants may contribute to hypoxia (lack of oxygen) in deep tissue by indiscriminately converting both normal oxygen and ROS molecules to water. As spin traps are reported to protect good oxygen by only attaching themselves to destructive free radicals, they could be considered superior. Research continues...

Formulation review

These few ingredients that are left are the possible actives and are highlighted in red.
Having learned about vitamins and antioxidants in the last sections, do you believe this cream can live up to it's anti-ageing and firming properties?

1. If the ingredients listed do not offer anti-ageing or firming effects, what skin conditions would they be most effective upon?

2. What ingredient mimics the bilayers of the stratum corneum?

3. What is the vitamin that works in synergy with tocopherol that is not present in the formula?

4. Are there any active ingredients that would indicate the quality of product?

5. Is this likely to be an expensive or modest retail product?

Ingredients: Aqua, Glycerine, Niacinamide, Cetyl alcohol, Propylene glycol, Petrolatum, Cyclopentasiloxane, Isopropyl palmitate, Panthenol, Tocopherol acetate, Tocopherol, Camellia sinensis, Ceramide 3, Stearyl alcohol, Myristyl alcohol, Propylene glycol stearate, Titanium dioxide, Palmitic acid, Stearic acid, Dimethicone, Carbomer, Steareth-21, Steareth-2, Disodium EDTA, Sodium hydroxide, Aluminim hydroxide, Phenoxyethanol, Imidazolidinyl urea, Methylparaben, Propylparaben, Benzyl alcohol, Parfum, Hexyl cinnamal, Linalool, Hydroxyisohexyl 3-cyclohexene carboxaldehyde, Butylphenol methylpropional, Alpha-isomethyl ionone, Hydroxycitronellal, Geraniol, Citronellol, Limonene.

Compatability check list

	Vitamin B group	Vitamin E group	Water soluble	Oil soluble	Melanogenesis inhibit	Epidermal support	Collagen fibril	Biomimetic	Occlusive	Antioxidant	Vitamin replacing	Restorative	Hydrating	Repair	Compromised skin
Niacinamide	✓		✓		✓	✓		✓		✓	✓	✓	✓	✓	✓
Panthenol	✓		✓			✓		✓		✓	✓	✓	✓	✓	✓
Tocopherol acetate		✓		✓		✓		✓		✓	✓	✓	✓	✓	✓
Tocopherol		✓		✓		✓		✓		✓	✓	✓	✓	✓	✓
Camellia sinensis			✓			✓		✓		✓			✓	✓	✓
	Ingredient specifications								Desirable criteria						

Sun protection actives & actions

Of all the cosmetic or skin care formulations applied to the skin, next to antioxidants, sun protection is without doubt the most important. Before we can even consider applying creams and lotions to reduce wrinkles, we must take steps to protect it from further damage.

The skins "built in" cellular protection systems gradually decline with age and the endogenous production of free radicals increase due to metabolic change.

We know our environment also plays an important role in the formation of superoxide radicals. UV radiation, ionizing radiation and pollutants, all promote the formation of these radicals.

All sun protection is not created equal, as various types of chemicals and compounds protect against different bands of UV radiation. We need to understand what the UV spectrum is and how it affects the skin, so that we can make more informed choices and educate our clients.

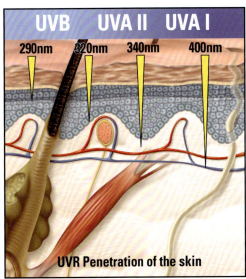

UVR Penetration of the skin

It is the UVR spectrum of 200nm to 400nm that demands the closest attention when referring to damaging radiation. To help make the UVR spectrum easier to understand, we have broken the spectrum down into a further 4 segments.

- UVC (200nm to 290nm)
- UVB (290nm to 320nm)
- UVA II (320nm to 340nm)
- UVA I (340nm to 400nm)

UVB penetrates the epidermis and is responsible for most epidermal cellular damage through its ability to create erythema and sunburn. It has been labelled the "tanning" ray because it stimulates the melanocyte to trigger melanogenesis. UVB was the part of the UV spectrum that historically commanded the most attention (UVA sun protection has only been pursued over the last 15 years) until it was realised that the UVA component of the spectrum was much more damaging to the connective tissue of the dermis.

UVA penetrates the skin to a greater depth than UVB, and is classified in further divisions of UVA II (320-340 nm) & UVA I (340-400 nm).

The relatively large amount of UVA and its ability to penetrate deeply into the skin (dermal layer) accounts for its greater significance when establishing cause of skin ageing by the increase in the collagenase enzyme that occurs with UVA exposure.

Recent studies have definitively established that UVA I is a causative factor in photo ageing. It is also the portion of the UVR spectrum most often associated with photosensitivities resulting from drugs, chemicals or disease.

What cellular damage occurs with UV radiation?

It has been inconclusively proven that the skin barrier defence system cells such as the langerhans cells, melanocytes and keratinocytes are affected by UVB radiation, with the langerhans cells especially sensitive to UVB, starting at just 0.5 of the minimal erythema dose (MED). This small dose of UVR can cause a decrease in both the total numbers of langerhans cells and their dendrite length, resulting in a reduction in the operation of skin barrier defence systems.

UVA II & I have the greatest penetration power, and have been linked to the damage of the collagen & elastin support fibres of the dermis. This is caused by an increase in the matrix metalloproteinases (MMP's) enzyme, collagenase. (Refer page 87 for more information)

UVC protection?

UVC is almost completely filtered out by the ozone layer, however if this changes in the future (as is often speculated), our knowledge and need for sun protection as we know it today, will really change.

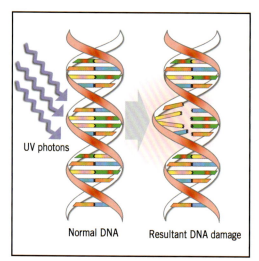

UV photons

Normal DNA   Resultant DNA damage

Sunburn induces oxidative stress and the resulting lipid peroxidation will compound and lead to mitochondria DNA damage of the epidermal cells. Protection from UVR is vital.

Sunburn can cause the vitamin A receptors found in a cell membrane to become inactive or to be reduced in number. Oxidisation of vitamin C will cause inactivity of vitamin E contributing to lipid peroxidation and a reduction in the overall health of epidermal cells, especially the keratinocyte.

This can result in atrophy of the spinosum layer contributing to irregular placement of melanin pigment, a reduction in skin barrier defence and an increase in TEWL (trans epidermal water loss).

What should a good sun protection product be able to do?

- Offer broad spectrum protection from sun burn.
- Contain an oil soluble antioxidant to reduce oxidative stress.
- Offer protection to the skin barrier defence system.
- Exhibit an anti-ageing protection profile.
- Exhibit a vitamin replacement profile (vitamins A,C & E).
- Enhance the skins own sun protection systems.

A suncare product that just prevents sunburn is not enough to ensure the skin will be cared for and premature ageing prevented.

Many domestic retail cosmetics designed for daily use have some, but not all of the protection systems that skin needs to protect it from sunburn and oxidative stress. Skin treatment therapy and appearance medicine products are far superior, because they contain skin care and sun-protection profiles, which address all levels and dangers of sun exposure.

All sun protection products and daily care cosmetics should ideally contain antioxidants. There are two predominant reasons why the skin may be overwhelmed by oxidative stress:

- Decreased effectiveness of protective enzyme systems.
- Increased radical exposure.

SPF Facts

SPF is not a true indicator of UVR protection factor, as it only relates to the UVB portion of the spectrum and at the time if writing this book, there is no uniform measure of UVA absorption.

Although there are broad-spectrum sunscreen products that protect against UVA and UVB radiation, it is important to remember that the SPF does not predict the level of UVA protection.

The discrepancy between sun protection effectiveness against sunburn and skin barrier defence protection has lead researchers to re-examine sun-protection strategies. Research is well advanced in laboratories around the world that formulate and supply beauty therapy products to our industry. The goal is to find substances that directly protect and support epidermal and dermal cells, and this is called biochemical protection.

Instead of just using high SPF UVR screening materials that protect against erythema, they have included antioxidants, cell repair/protection, hydration/skin lipid support, and DNA repair agents to reduce cell damage.

Sun protection methodologies

There are two types of sun protection products. One type reflects the UV rays (known as physical or particulate) and the other type that absorbs and converts UV rays (termed chemical).

Of all the currently used sun protection chemicals available, only one physical block (zinc oxide) has the ability to offer complete broad-spectrum protection. Many of the chemical absorption types are only effective in the UVB range, with very few with the ability to cover both UVA I & II.

This is why a quality formulation usually employs a number of different overlapping types to cover the full spectrum. Many cosmetic products. including moisturisers and make-up now contain sun protection ingredients; some not only to protect the user, but also to protect other UV sensitive ingredients in the formulation, just as a preservative does.

Physical sun protection

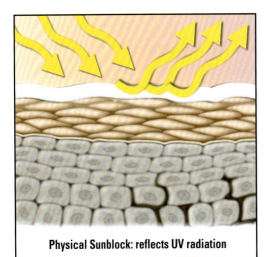

Physical Sunblock: reflects UV radiation

As a result of their reflective abilities, physical screens offer broad-spectrum protection (UVA & B).

Physical sun protection contain tiny particles of either metals or earth-based reflectors suspended in an oily film. Recent developments with physical sun protection include micronisation of the particles and the experimentation with the coating of the particles with teflon, mica and silk to produce a smoother feel. Formulators are now challenged to develop sun protection products to meet the requirements of growing consumer demand for broad-spectrum protection and high SPF values. To achieve high SPF and broad-spectrum protection, a mixture of chemical and physical UV filters have been used in combination.

Titanium dioxide (TiO2)

TiO2 is one of the 21 FDA approved sun protection chemicals with an approved usage level of 2 to 25%. A physical block that remains on the skin surface scattering and reflecting UVR. Its usage within the skin care industry is dependant on molecular size. The smaller the particle size, the more unobtrusive its application. Large particles cause mild skin whitening on some skins. Using words like "micro" or ultra" in marketing is in reference to particle size.

Zinc oxide (ZnO)

Has an effective physical blocking property, now in a micro-fine formulation that eliminates whitening. Physical sun protection are less likely to be totally waterproof, as there are difficulties in manufacturing truly waterproof oil-in-water formulations with the physical screening agents. Physical sun protection containing zinc oxide or titanium dioxide protect against UVB and UVA. However, zinc oxide blocks more UV radiation than titanium dioxide and, therefore, is the preferred ingredient (refer to comparison chart on page 88).

Encapsulated micro fine zinc oxide using nanoparticles

Micro-fine zinc oxide has been increasingly used since 1997, when the US FDA approved it as a safe and effective UV filter for personal care products. Since then, a novel water dispersible, broad-spectrum sun protection has been developed. It consists of nanoparticles of micro-fine zinc oxide encapsulated by octyl triazone and octyl methoxycinnamate (Sunzerse®). Octyl triazone has special interest in its own right as it exhibits the highest UVB absorption of all chemical sun protection available. This type of sun protection is a good example of a modern, dual technology approach.

Nanomaterials used in sun protection products

We discussed nano-technology in the earlier chapter on cosmetic formulation delivery systems. We will now look at this new nano-material in the field of sun protection. A nanoparticle is an object having three external dimensions on the nano-scale. Here the nano-scale is being defined as approximately 1-100nm.

The inorganic sun protection titanium dioxide and zinc oxide are perhaps the most common type of nanoparticle in personal care, and one of the debates is whether or not TiO2 or Zn is in fact a nano-material, so this must first be examined.

It is known that the properties of scattering and absorption of UV are measurable and results can vary by particle size and refractive index.

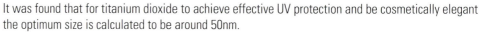

Aggregate:

A particle comprised of strongly bonded or fused particles, wherein the resulting external surface area, may be significantly smaller than the sum of calculated surface areas of the individual components.

Agglomerate:

A collection of loosely bound particles or aggregates or mixtures of the two wherein the resulting external surface area is similar to the sum of the surface areas of the individual components.

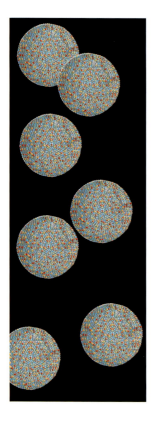

It was found that for titanium dioxide to achieve effective UV protection and be cosmetically elegant the optimum size is calculated to be around 50nm.

Many suppliers of fine particle titanium dioxide offer different particle sizes (10nm to over 100nm) resulting in confusion. The answer to this, lies in understanding that a particle can have an external size greater than the nano-scale, but consists of aggregates or agglomerates of smaller particles that are within the nano-scale range.

Fine particle titanium dioxide is manufactured as nanoparticles that are typically 10-20 nm in size, and some suppliers are marketing this as the particle size. Not so. These nanoparticles form tightly bound aggregates (see definition side bar), which have a larger size. These aggregates (the smallest particles) will join together to form loosely bound agglomerates, that have a particle size greater than 1 micron, placing them well out of the nano-scale range.

The, as yet, unanswered question is to what degree the agglomerates break down, and what the particle size is in the final formulation.

While the debate continues over whether the "particle size" of inorganic sun protection are nanomaterials or not, the question of safety should be answered.

Some of the concerns came from size and others were based on whether or not they had been tested properly to ensure safety.

For this discussion we will stay within the boundaries of sun protection and it must be remembered that fine particle grades of TiO_2 and ZnO have been around for nearly 20 years and have been extensively tested (and used). To be effective and cosmetically acceptable TiO_2 needs to be no smaller than 50nm and this size has been available and in use for some time.

The question I ask is: what benefit is there in a sun-protection chemical being able to reach the basal layer and transverse the dermal/epidermal junction? The cells and systems it is supposed to protect are the keratinocyte and the epidermis as a whole. In addition to this, using any sort of sun protection factor only prevents erythema; they do not prevent cell damage. Only antioxidants are able to do this with the current level of technology. Perhaps some formulators need to go back to basics and consider the objective of effective sun protection.

Nanospheres prevent sun protection chemicals from oxidation?

Sun protection chemicals are used to protect skin from UV radiation. When this happens, many sun protection molecules are reactive towards UV radiation and undergo isomerization or decomposition (a type of chemical oxidation). This depletes the concentration of the protective molecules in the skin and the efficiency of the sun protection is reduced. This is just one reason for re-application of your sun protection cream. Various strategies are being developed in the industry to deliver and protect the sun protection molecules. One of these strategies is the use of nano-encapsulation using poly (D,L-Lactide) microspheres. By loading nanoparticles with a sun protection chemical such as octyl methoxycinnamate (OMC) a formulation will be more effective over a longer period of time, with improved photostability as a result of the nano-encapsulation.

Micronised reflecting powders (a new subclass of physical sun protection)

Unlike the traditional zinc and titanium dioxide reflecting particulates, the newer micronised reflecting powders may offer a solution for those skins that cannot tolerate traditional sun protection creams. Silica microspheres, micronised talc and nylon powders designed to reflect light, are being commonly found in make-up that exhibits a broad spectrum sun protection factor.

These micronised powders are generally tinted to render them almost invisible on application.

Chemical sun protection

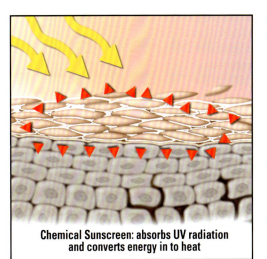

Chemical Sunscreen: absorbs UV radiation and converts energy in to heat

The majority of sun protection compounds available are chemical UV absorbers. As previously described, these compounds absorb and convert UV energy into heat that is dispersed by the skins surface. Chemical sun protection are classified commercially by their main chemical types:

- Para amino benzoates (PABA derivatives)
- Cinnamates
- Benzophenones
- Anthranilates
- Dibenzoylmethanes
- Imidazoles
- Salicylates

Para amino benzoates (UVB)

PABA (para-aminobenzoic acid) was one of the first widely used chemical types, however rarely used today because of irritation and solubility problems. Chemists however, have developed many derivatives of this substance known as para amino benzoates, with some manufacturers using these derivatives and claiming their formulations are PABA free.

This is somewhat of a misleading statement, and the therapist must be vigilant when recommending a PABA free sun protection to a client who may be allergic to PABA. An example of this misinformation is a product called Padimate-O, which is really Octyl Dimethyl PABA.

- Amino benzoic acid
- Glyceryl amino benzoate
- Ethyl-4-bis amino benzoate
- Amyl dimethyl PABA
- Glyceryl PABA
- Ethyl dihydroxypropyl PABA
- Octyl dimethyl PABA (2-ethylhexyl dimethyl PABA)

Salicylates (UVB)

This group of compounds were the replacements for PABA formulations and are based on an aspirin-like substance.

- Octyl salicylate (2-ethylhexyl salicylate)
- Homosalate (HMS or homomenthyl salicylate)
- Triethanolamine salicylate

Cinnamates (UVB)

The cinnamate family are the most frequently used UVB absorbers in the United States. They are often found in colour cosmetics that have an SPF factor.

- 2-Ethoxyethyl-p-Methoxy cinnamate
- Diethanolamine-p-methoxy cinnamate
- Octyl-p-methoxy cinnamate (2-ethylhexyl-p-methoxy cinnamate)

Benzophenones (UVA)

This group of organic UVA compounds are also used as the UV protectors of formulations.

- Avobenzone (Butyl methoxy-dibenzoylmethane)
- Dioxybenzone(Benzophenone-8)
- Oxybenzone (Benzophone-3)
- Sulisobenzone (Benzophenone-4)
- Dihydroxybenzophenene (Benzophenone-1)
- Tetrahydroxybenzophenone (Benzophenone-2)
- Octabenzone (Benzophenone-12)
- 2,2-Dihydroxy-4,4-dimethoxy benzophenone (Benzophenone-6)

before application can often provide the best results, keeping in mind that the blending of the two products is likely to reduce the SPF rating due to dilution. The easy fix for this of course is to use a sun protection with a higher SPF.

Sun protection dosage

One of the most important aspects of understanding sun protection products and their correct use is to fully comprehend the relationship between sun exposure and afforded protection by the product. Many sun protection users believe the myth that if they wear sun protection they are fully protected from UV exposure and the suns harmful UVA and UVB rays and will not burn. An equally subscribed myth is that re-application will increase burn time by the same factor as initial application.
Of course, both of these statements are indeed myths, however it is perhaps the second statement that is the most misunderstood. The explaination and chart below illustrates this occurrence more graphically.

Let us consider a scenario where an individual with an unprotected burn time of 4 minutes, applies a sun protection with a 30 SPF rating. In ideal best circumstances without re-application, sunburn or 100% MED (Minimal erythema dose) will occur after approx. 120 minutes.

Then, if this individual re-applies another coat of 30 SPF after just 60 minutes, the rate of burn will indeed be slowed, but it will not provide another 120 minutes of protection. Why? This is because after the first 60 minutes, approx. 50% of the individuals MED would have already been received.
The re-application, rather than re-setting the exposure time back to zero, instead acts as a "booster" to the initial application. (This is important and where most people miscalculate remaining burn time)

After the next 60 minutes, (Total 120 minutes sun exposure) the "boosting" effect of the re-application will mean the individual has received approximately another 25% of their MED, and if no futher re-application occurs, they will reach 100% MED at approximately 150 minutes from the start time. On the other hand, if sunscreen is re-applied again at the 120-minute mark, the final 25% of MED will be used up at approx. 165 minutes from initial exposure. What this means is that with two re-applications of sunscreen at the 60 and 120 minute marks, only 45 minutes more "safe" time of sun exposure is afforded, than provided by a single application.

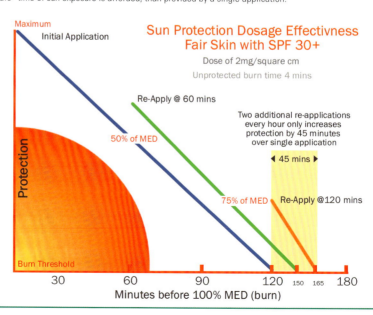

Why should a phototype 4 and higher use sun protection?

Skins that are classified as "high risk for pigmentation" are those that have the ability to tan easily with a phototype of four, five and six.

Although these skin colours may not burn easily, they have the ability to develop pigmented lesions very easily (especially post-inflammatory pigmentation).

Therefore, long hours of unprotected sun exposure should be avoided by wearing a low SPF sun protection product that includes antioxidants that slow down melanogenesis (e.g. magnesium ascorbyl phosphate and ßeta-carotene).

On the following page you will find a quick reference guide to popular sun protection compounds and their respective coverage of the UVR spectrum. It includes both physical and chemical types.

A brief word on UV damage and collagenase

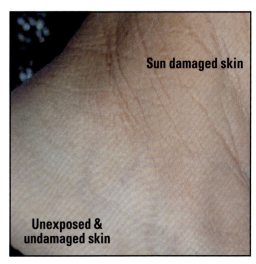

Sun damaged skin

Unexposed & undamaged skin

Solar Exposure Comparison

This photo is an example of a 59 year old, phototype 2 skin tone with the red head gene (MC1R). The lower neckline has always been protected from sun exposure, and shows as a beautifully textured, unlined and unmarked skin. The upper neckline is showing a skin that has all of the hallmarks of an ageing sun damaged skin, and proves the effects of sun exposure.

Maintenance is a critical aspect of any normal tissue development and repair, this is achieved by a constant two-way communication with the cells embedded within it or surrounding it.

Regulated turnover of dermal structures like collagen and elastin is achieved through the interplay of two enzymes called collagenase and elastase.

These enzymes are important in regular maintainance and replacement, including the repair of dermal tissue during wound healing.

These enzymes are very potent when active, and it has been recently determined that ultraviolet radiation (UVR) activates a protein complex called AP-1, which activates the production of large amounts of collagenase and elastase (MMP's) enzymes.

These enzymes are regulated by built in defense systems known as TIMPs that loose effectivness with age, resulting in even exposure to small amounts of UVR (such as every other day) enough to induce sustained MMP production at high levels.

When this happens the collagenase and elastase enzymes begin to break down the very fibres they were designed to protect, contributing to a breakdown of the dermal matrix and skin ageing.

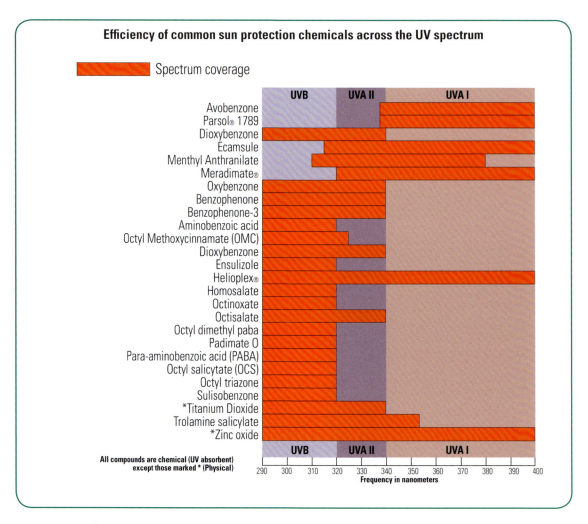

Efficiency of common sun protection chemicals across the UV spectrum

Spectrum coverage

(Chart: compounds listed vertically — Avobenzone, Parsol 1789, Dioxybenzone, Ecamsule, Menthyl Anthranilate, Meradimate, Oxybenzone, Benzophenone, Benzophenone-3, Aminobenzoic acid, Octyl Methoxycinnamate (OMC), Dioxybenzone, Ensulizole, Helioplex, Homosalate, Octinoxate, Octisalate, Octyl dimethyl paba, Padimate O, Para-aminobenzoic acid (PABA), Octyl salicytate (OCS), Octyl triazone, Sulisobenzone, *Titanium Dioxide, Trolamine salicylate, *Zinc oxide — plotted across UVB, UVA II, UVA I)

All compounds are chemical (UV absorbent) except those marked * (Physical)

Frequency in nanometers: 290 300 310 320 330 340 350 360 370 380 390 400

Overuse of sun protection products

A reduction in efficiency of skin barrier defence systems and vitamin D deficiency can be caused by the overuse of sun protection products that exhibit very high sun protection factors (SPF).

We know that part of the skin's natural defence system is the melanogenesis process, and when the melanocytes remain inactive for long periods of time, they become less able to respond quickly when required.

Similarly, vitamin D deficiency can occur when sun protection is "overworn" to the point where virtually no 7-dehydrocholesterol conversion from UV exposure occurs. When you consider that around 80 per cent of our vitamin D comes from exposure to the sun, the only alternative is supplements and dietary intake.

While there is truth in the fact that a higher SPF will offer a higher level of protection, you must consider if you really need it. If you spend most of the day indoors, and drive to and from work before 9am and after 5pm, there is very little chance that you will get sunburnt and suffer cellular damage.

A sensible balance of sun exposure and sun protection can ensure against vitamin D deficiency without being at risk of skin cancer. The recommended amount of sunlight each day is a few minutes of sunlight exposure before 10am and after 3pm each day and two to three hours of sunlight exposure over the week.

Formulation review

In the final review of this formulation in this section of the book, you will be looking at sun protection actives. We can see here the lone remaining ingredient is our sun protection.
It may have a dual purpose however, as the white compound used can have the effect of making the skin appear brighter/whiter upon application.
The other obvious function is that of a colouring, to make the cream appear more pleasing and less opaque.

This product has been marketed as an anti-ageing product, with an emphasis on the reduction of wrinkles. You may have already reached the conclusion that for the reduction of wrinkles, the composition may fall short of marketing and customer expectations because of the combination of ingredients. It may however, offer some protection from the elements of day to day living and at best, function as a simple day cream of average standard (and consequently command an average price).

Section two of this book will deal more specifically with the types of ingredients that have an effect on specific skin conditions. This will help you further identify the types of ingredients that will provide particular actions.

Ingredients: Aqua, Glycerine, Niacinamide, Cetyl alcohol, Propylene glycol, Petrolatum, Cyclopentasiloxane, Isopropyl palmitate, Panthenol, Tocopherol acetate, Tocopherol, Camellia sinensis, Ceramide 3, Stearyl alcohol, Myristyl alcohol, Propylene glycol stearate, Titanium dioxide, Palmitic acid, Stearic acid, Dimethicone, Carbomer, Steareth-21, Steareth-2, Disodium EDTA, Sodium hydroxide, Aluminim hydroxide, Phenoxyethanol, Imidazolidinyl urea, Methylparaben, Propylparaben, Benzyl alcohol, Parfum, Hexyl cinnamal, Linalool, Hydroxyisohexyl 3-cyclohexene carboxaldehyde, Butylphenol methylpropional, Alpha-isomethyl ionone, Hydroxycitronellal, Geraniol, Citronellol, Limonene.

Compatability check list

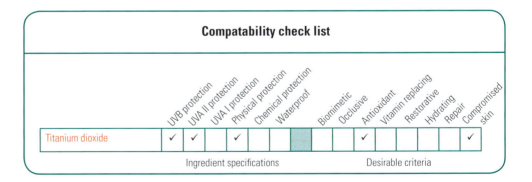

	UVB protection	UVA II protection	UVA I protection	Physical protection	Chemical protection	Waterproof	Biomimetic	Occlusive	Antioxidant	Vitamin replacing	Restorative	Hydrating	Repair	Compromised skin
Titanium dioxide	✓	✓		✓				✓						✓

Ingredient specifications   Desirable criteria

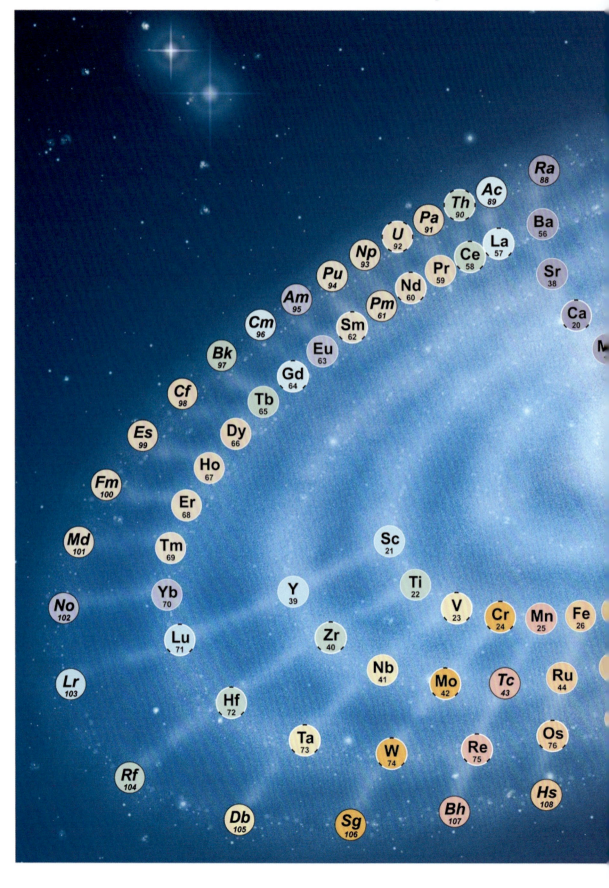

The periodic table of the elements

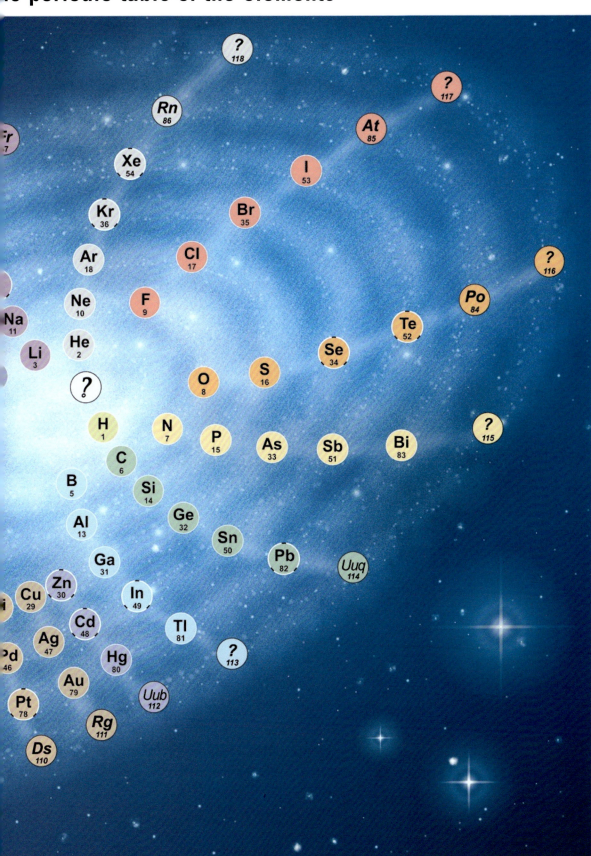

Listing of table of elements over the page

References:
P J Stewart, 'A new Image of the Periodic Table', Education in Chemistry, 41 (6), 156-158, November 2004.

P J Stewart, 'A Century on from Dmitrii Mendeleev: Tables and Spirals, Noble Gases and Nobel Prizes', Foundations of Chemistry, 9 (3), pp.235-245, October 2007.

Periodic table of the elements

SYMB.	NAME	No.	R.A.M.	SYMB.	NAME	No.	R.A.M.
Ac	Actinium	89	(227)	N	Nitrogen	7	14.007
Ag	Silver	47	107.87	Na	Sodium	11	22.990
Al	Aluminium	13	26.982	Nb	Niobium	41	92.906
Am	Americium	95	(243)	Nd	Neodymium	60	144.24
	Antimony: *see Sb*			Ne	Neon	10	20.180
Ar	Argon	18	39.948	n	Neutronium	0	1.0087
As	Arsenic	33	74.922	Ni	Nickel	28	58.693
At	Astatine	85	(210)	No	Nobelium	102	(259)
Au	Gold	79	196.97	Np	Neptunium	93	237.05
B	Boron	5	10.811	O	Oxygen	8	15.999
Ba	Barium	56	137.33	Os	Osmium	76	190.23
Be	Beryllium	4	9.0122	P	Phosphorus	15	30.974
Bh	Bohrium	107	(262)	Pa	Protactinium	91	231.04
Bi	Bismuth	83	208.98	Pb	Lead	82	207.20
Bk	Berkelium	97	(247)	Pd	Palladium	46	106.42
Br	Bromine	35	79.904	Pm	Promethium	61	(145)
C	Carbon	6	12.011	Po	Polonium	84	(209)
Ca	Calcium	20	40.078		Potassium: *see K*		
Cd	Cadmium	48	112.41	Pr	Praseodymium	59	140.91
Ce	Cerium	58	140.12	Pt	Platinum	78	195.08
Cf	Californium	98	(251)	Pu	Plutonium	94	(244)
Cl	Chlorine	17	35.453	Ra	Radium	88	(226)
Cm	Curium	96	(247)	Rb	Rubidium	37	85.468
Co	Cobalt	27	58.933	Re	Rhenium	75	186.21
Cr	Chromium	24	51.996	Rf	Rutherfordium	104	(261)
Cs	Caesium	55	132.91	Rg	Roentgenium	111	(272)
Cu	Copper	29	63.546	Rh	Rhodium	45	102.91
Db	Dubnium	105	(262)	Rn	Radon	86	(222)
Ds	Darmstadtium	110	(271)	Ru	Ruthenium	44	101.07
Dy	Dysprosium	66	162.50	S	Sulphur	16	32.065
Er	Erbium	68	167.26	Sb	Antimony	51	121.76
Es	Einsteinium	99	(254)	Sc	Scandium	21	44.996
Eu	Europium	63	151.97	Se	Selenium	34	78.960
F	Fluorine	9	18.998	Sg	Seaborgium	106	(266)
Fe	Iron	26	55.845	Si	Silicon	14	28.086
Fm	Fermium	100	(257)		Silver: *see Ag*		
Fr	Francium	87	(223)	Sm	Samarium	62	150.36
Ga	Gallium	31	69.723	Sn	Tin	50	118.71
Gd	Gadolinium	64	157.25		Sodium: *see Na*		
Ge	Germanium	32	72.640	Sr	Strontium	38	87.620
	Gold: *see Au*			Ta	Tantalum	73	180.95
H	Hydrogen	1	1.0079	Tb	Terbium	65	158.93
He	Helium	2	4.0026	Tc	Technetium	43	(99)
Hf	Hafnium	72	178.49	Te	Tellurium	52	127.60
Hg	Mercury	80	200.59	Th	Thorium	90	232.04
Ho	Holmium	67	164.93	Ti	Titanium	22	47.867
Hs	Hassium	108	(265)		Tin: see Sn		
I	Iodine	53	126.90	Tl	Thallium	81	204.38
In	Indium	49	114.82	Tm	Thulium	69	168.93
Ir	Iridium	77	192.22		Tungsten: *see W*		
	Iron: *see Fe*			U	Uranium	92	238.03
K	Potassium	19	39.098	Uub	Ununbium	112	(277)
Kr	Krypton	36	83.800	Uuq	Ununquadium	114	(289)
La	Lanthanum	57	138.91	V	Vanadium	23	50.942
	Lead: *see Pb*			W	Tungsten	74	183.84
Li	Lithium	3	6.9410	Xe	Xenon	54	131.29
Lr	Lawrencium	103	(260)	Y	Yttrium	39	88.906
Lu	Lutetium	71	174.97	Yb	Ytterbium	70	173.04
Md	Mendelevium	101	(258)	Zn	Zinc	30	65.390
	Mercury: *see Hg*			Zr	Zirconium	40	91.224
Mg	Magnesium	12	24.305				
Mn	Manganese	25	54.938				
Mo	Molybdenum	42	95.940				
Mt	Meitnerium	109	(266)				

Chapter Two

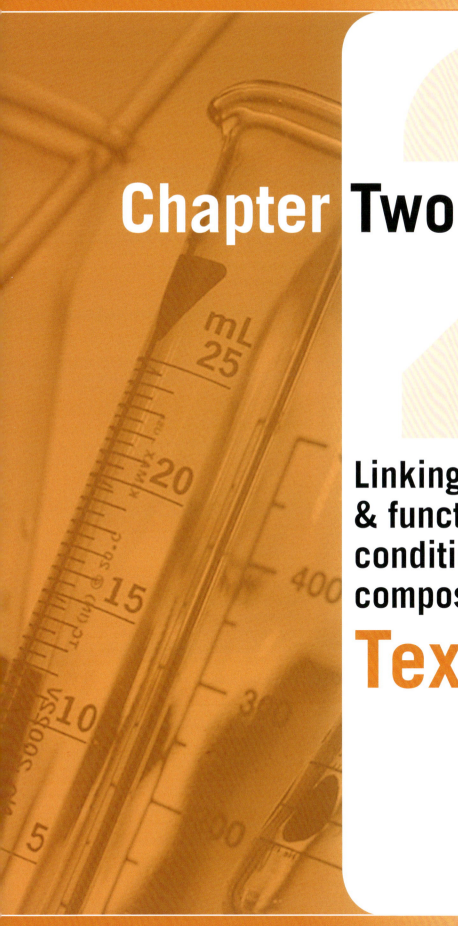

Linking skin structure & function to skin condition & product composition

Texture

Linking skin structure & function to skin condition & product composition

All of the skin conditions a practising therapist diagnoses and treats every day will fall into one or more of three categories. These three categories are known as Texture, Colour and Secretion and are controlled or influenced by two major factors: intrinsic and extrinsic.

The first is the intrinsic factor & genetics of basic majority skin type, skin colour and the risk factors associated with that skin colour.
The second is the extrinsic factor such as diet, lifestyle, environment, medication, illness, and of course skin care products used. The diagnostic pathway below illustrates this.
Both the intrinsic and extrinsic factors of the skin are found in the consultation process. Linking these leading causes to the damaged or influenced cells and systems that are behind a skin condition is fundamental to the Pastiche Method® of skin analysis.

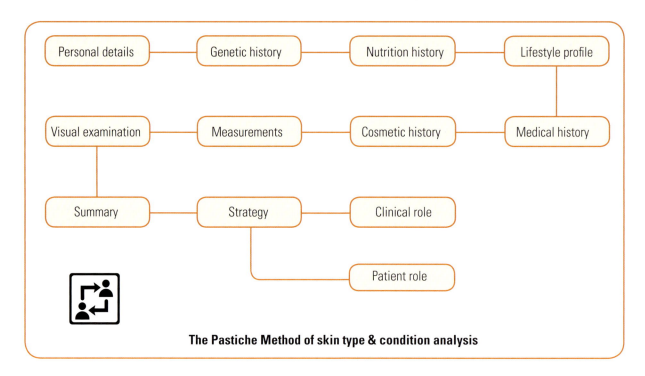

The Pastiche Method of skin type & condition analysis

There are two elements of planning a treatment program and choosing the right modality and chemicals needed for corrective intervention or treatment of a skin condition.
The first is the linking of skin condition to skin structure and function, and the second is to link product composition to skin structure and function.

There is a synergy, pattern and a flow to this method, and it is based on the biological events and chemical reality rather than marketing hype. Following this path in a logical manner will ensure that you will always choose the most appropriate treatment protocols and approach.

This flow chart will remind us of the Pastiche Method protocols that need to be part of planning a treatment program. If the protocols are not followed, success will be severely compromised.

Basic majority skin type	Protocol during in salon treatment
Lipid Dry	Use cleanser & toner for dry skin Maintain acid mantle at all times Use non drying masks Do not use harsh abrasive exfoliants Extreme care with chemical peels Moderate use of vapour zone Massage with essential fatty acids or high emollient slip cream Complete treatment with an occlusive cream
Permanent diffused redness	Use cleanser & toner with no fragrance or colour Avoid extremes of hot & cold Avoid over vaso-dilation of capillaries Maintain acid mantle at all times Use non drying masks Do not use harsh abrasive exfoliants Extreme care with chemical peels (If at all) Use cool spray or Lucas Championnière Massage with essential fatty acids Complete treatment with an occlusive cream
Oily	Use cleansers & toners for oily skin If acneic use cleanser & toner without fragrance or colour Maintain acid mantle at all times Only use masks for oily skin on oily areas Do not use harsh abrasive exfoliants Moderate use of vaporzone machine (Or use Lucas Championnière)

In addition to being aware of the protocols of basic majority skin type, the clinician must also practice the protocols for treating a phototype 3 to 6 skin colour that has the intrinsic tendency of "high risk" for pigmentation and scarring.

High risk for pigmentation during a salon treatment	
Phototypes 3 to 6 will have the predisposition to be at high risk". Always check the genetics, tanning ability and sun burn history of a client.	High risk of hyper/hypo-pigmentation after Laser/IPL treatment. Check melanin density on the treatment site before every treatment. This reading should always be referenced back to the original melanin average reading taken at the consultation or patch test appointment. High risk for trauma, heat & chemically caused pigmentation, & moderate risk for all other pigmented skin conditions.

Skin barrier defence systems

It is appropriate that we review the skin barrier defence systems at this point because the ability of any topically applied formulations to perform their respective actions will be determined by its ability to transverse these barrier defence systems. If specific features of a formulation are not met, the likelihood of the active ingredients reaching their targeted site is greatly minimised.

The skin has a number of lines of defence against penetration of foreign objects and substances, essentially rendering the skin resistant to absorption of substances the body considers alien. The three main barriers are defined as the natural microflora, the epidermal barrier, and finally the immune system, with a number of sub-systems within each:

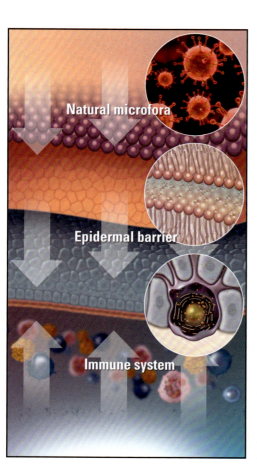

Acid mantle
The first line of skin barrier defence is the acid mantle, with a pH of 5.5. This acidic environment in which micro flora/bacteria resides contribute to the inhibition of more harmful bacteria.

Stratum corneum
Keratinocyte has differentiated into a corneocyte. The hydrophobic corneocyte repels water and is embedded in bilayers of oil and water. (Bilayers)

Bi-layers (Ceramides)
The lipid barrier is formed by the differentiation of the keratinocyte, from which comes the lipid-enriched contents of the epidermal odland bodies. These lipids exist in the intercellular spaces of the stratum corneum, governing the permeability of the epidermis and contributing to cell adhesion of the stratum corneum while helping slow TEWL.

Granular layer
The granular layer is an effective barrier that helps to prevent the absorption of many substances. It also slows down trans-epidermal water flow, retaining water in the lower cell-dividing layer. (Basal layer)

Cell membranes
For the skin's natural protection systems to function at optimum levels, all cells that contribute to that protection system must have a healthy and permeable membrane.

Langerhans cell (LC's)
An active system of skin immune defence protects the skin against external attacks; LC's are the essential cells of this system in association with keratinocytes.

Melanogenesis (formation of the pigment melanin)
An integral part of skin and cell barrier defence against ultra violet radiation. (UVR)

Dermal/epidermal junction (Basal lamina)
A permeable barrier between epidermis and dermis. The basal lamina serves as a structural support for tissues and as a permeability barrier to regulate movement of both cell and molecules.

Lymphatic system
The lymph and blood vessels have the function of keeping the composition and amount of fluids in our system constant, while working with all skin barrier defence systems.

Linking skin structure and function to product compostion

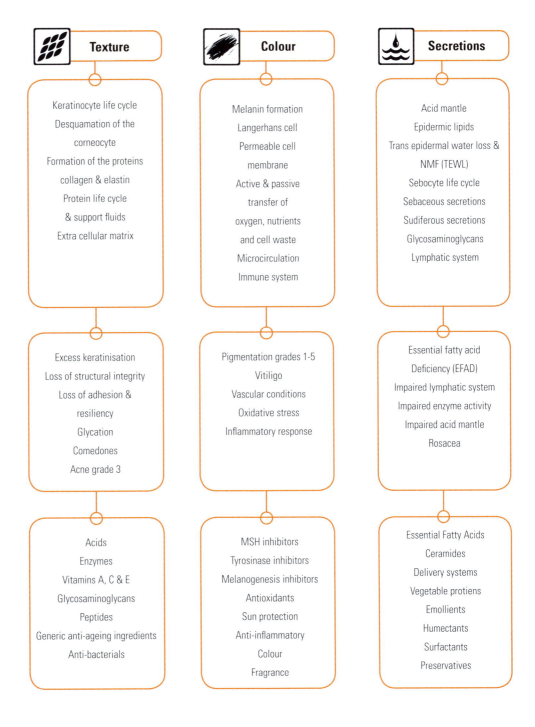

Texture

Keratinocyte life cycle
Desquamation of the
corneocyte
Formation of the proteins
collagen & elastin
Protein life cycle
& support fluids
Extra cellular matrix

Excess keratinisation
Loss of structural integrity
Loss of adhesion &
resiliency
Glycation
Comedones
Acne grade 3

Acids
Enzymes
Vitamins A, C & E
Glycosaminoglycans
Peptides
Generic anti-ageing ingredients
Anti-bacterials

Colour

Melanin formation
Langerhans cell
Permeable cell
membrane
Active & passive
transfer of
oxygen, nutrients
and cell waste
Microcirculation
Immune system

Pigmentation grades 1-5
Vitiligo
Vascular conditions
Oxidative stress
Inflammatory response

MSH inhibitors
Tyrosinase inhibitors
Melanogenesis inhibitors
Antioxidants
Sun protection
Anti-inflammatory
Colour
Fragrance

Secretions

Acid mantle
Epidermic lipids
Trans epidermal water loss &
NMF (TEWL)
Sebocyte life cycle
Sebaceous secretions
Sudiferous secretions
Glycosaminoglycans
Lymphatic system

Essential fatty acid
Deficiency (EFAD)
Impaired lymphatic system
Impaired enzyme activity
Impaired acid mantle
Rosacea

Essential Fatty Acids
Ceramides
Delivery systems
Vegetable protiens
Emollients
Humectants
Surfactants
Preservatives

Skin conditions that change the texture of skin

Two factors control the texture of the skin; one that influences the epidermis or external factors and the other the dermis or internal factors. By separating the skin into these two categories, the cells and systems of each are addressed separately to help make them easier to understand.

Epidermal

The renewal and desquamation of the stratum corneum is the external factor, and is responsible for the **external** appearance (smoothness, regularity) of the skin. When the desquamation of the skin is impaired or abnormal, there is a build up of dead cells which can appear either as a simple skin condition needing exfoliation, through to chronic skin disorder, such as psoriasis.
When these conditions are present, the surface texture and appearance of the skin undergoes change.

Dermal

The process of cellular renewal and connective tissue formation in the papillary and reticular layers of the dermis are also responsible for the outward appearance and texture of the skin.
It is here that the structural integrity, or the form of the soft tissue, is determined by the presence of collagen and elastin. These are the **internal** factors. It is in the lower layers that the most cellular activity occurs, and consequently the therapist must think about the effects any treatments will ultimately have on the cellular division and the primary functions of these layers.

Skin conditions related to texture

- Hyper-keratinisation
- Open comedones (Non inflammatory acne grade 2)
- Closed comedones (Non inflammatory acne grade 1)
- Inflammatory acne grade 3
- Collagens loss of integrity & thin skin density

Cells and systems involved or influenced

- Keratinocyte
- Fibroblast
- Sebocyte life cycle
- Sebaceous gland
- Collagen fibril
- Glycosaminoglycans

Effective chemicals/actives

- Acids
- Antibacterial
- Vitamin C
- Vitamin B
- Growth factors
- Androgen inhibitors
- Enzymes
- Vitamin A
- Bioflavonoids
- Peptides

For information on the complete lifecycle of keratinocyte, read pages
24 to 29 in the book
Advanced Skin Analysis
ISBN 978-0-476-00665-2

Skin condition: Hyper-keratinisation

Key points of the keratinocyte life cycle:

The keratinocyte is the primary cell of the epidermis and is responsible for generating and maintaining the skin barrier defence systems of the epidermis. During it's life cycle, (differentiation) this cell will undergo change many times to produce these defence systems.

In the spinosum layer, keratin filaments called desmosomes join the keratinocytes to one another and these are responsible for cell-to-cell adhesion and strength of the epidermis. In the granular layer these keratin filaments will dissolve with the help of hydrophilic enzymes (glycosidase and protease) and prepare the cell for desquamation.
When these desmosomes do not dissolve efficiently the keratinocyte cells remain attached to each other and cause skin congestion and hyper keratinisation.

Contributing to the skin barrier defence systems is the resulting formation of mature, flexible corneocytes embedded in the bilayers that has been secreted by differentiating keratinocytes just before termination of the cornification process.
The corneocytes are embedded in bilayers of oil and water the oil phase being primarily ceramides. When the keratinocyte is unable to make high percentages of ceramides, (Due to EFAD) poor desquamation and fast evaporation of water will result. In addition, the sebaceous and sudiferous secretions will not be emulsified into a complete functioning acid mantle.

Cause and effect on cells and systems:

Thinking three dimensionally is the key, remembering to visualise the life cycle of the keratinocyte and related cells and systems of the epidermis. Asking yourself the question: "what does this cell require to function efficiently and correctly"? "What would happen if those requirements were not in place"? Once you determine the effect and cellular damage, you will then be able to put a corrective program for clinic and home care in place.

Primary causes and affect on cells & systems that contribute to hyper-keratinisation

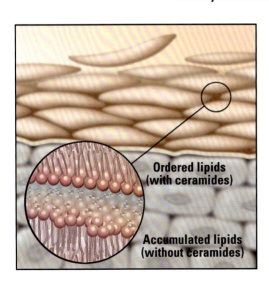

During differentiation, the keratinocyte will undergo change many times.

Ordered lipids (with ceramides)

Accumulated lipids (without Ceramides)

- A lack of free water or low humidity will impair the enzymes required for the dissolution of tethering desmosomes, resulting in poor desquamation of cell.

- A lack of free water prevents the alignment of the epidermal bilayer lipids.

- EFAD will cause poor alignment of bilayers, resulting in sticky corneocytes.

- EFAD will result in poor quality or quantity of ceramides and bilayers, causing lipids to accumulate into small balls, contributing toward the formation of milia. (See image at left)

- EFAD will result in lower quantities of ceramides, which are the emulsifiers of the acid mantle. Sebaceous & sudiferous secretions are unable to mix without ceramide emulsifiers.

- Skin with psoriasis or keratosis pilaris history have a tendency to hyper-keratinisation. Always check consultation details.

Skin condition: Open & closed comedones

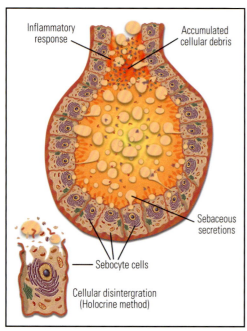

Essential fatty acids are vital for high quality and quantity of sebaceous secretions

The primary causes of this non inflammatory acne is excess keratinisation (As previously discussed) and an accumulation of cellular debris within the sebaceous glands.

This debris is produced as a by-product of poor quality sebocyte cell membranes, which may be due to essential fatty acid deficiency.

When the sebocyte is in good health, it produces primarily triglycerides, (50%) which are an important component of the acid mantle, free fatty acids and the resultant 5.5 pH required to maintain skin barrier defence systems.

Key points of the sebocyte life-cycle

The sebocyte has a life-cycle of 14-20 days, and during its journey from mitosis to the sebaceous gland interior, the sebocyte will breakdown as much of itself as possible into sebaceous gland oil.

The final expression of the sebaceous lipids by the holocrine method of secretion should result in a large amount of oil and a small amount of cellular debris. If however, the sebocyte was not in optimum health, a small amount of oil and a large amount of cellular debris may result.

This will ultimately lead to blocking of the sebaceous gland exit and the beginning of micro comedones. Further, if the skin has a basic majority type of oily with large amounts of cellular debris, including poor quality oil, then a more severe condition of acne and comedones could result.

Substances to be avoided with oily acneic skins:

- Steroids
- Testosterone
- Free Fatty Acids (In cosmetic formulations)
- Chlorine, tar and other petro-chemical compounds
- Synthetic red or orange pigments (DC Reds are comedogenic)

- Ultraviolet Radiation
- Barbiturates

- Harsh drying substances
- Amphetamines
- High humidity/humectants

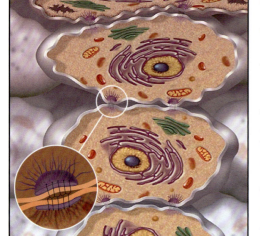

Tethering desmosomes are dissolved with acids

Choosing a methodology

What always needs to be considered when choosing a methodology of treatment is the basic majority skin type, phototype risk factors, phototype skin colour, and the contraindications/protocols that are standard for these factors.

So often a methodology is touted to be "suitable for all skin types", but what is often not taken into consideration are the accompanying risks and contraindications specific to intrinsic skin type and phototype.
The same considerations and contraindications should also be applied to the extrinsic skin conditions.

This is particularly relevant when choosing a methodology for hyper-keratinisation and comedones, because the chemicals most effective in addressing the dissolution of desmosomes and corneo-desmosomes are acids and enzymes.

Treatment solutions for hyper keratinisation & comedones

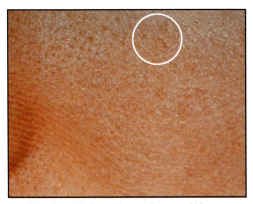

Hyper keratinisation with poor alignment of bilayers

Before using acids and enzymes it is imperative to ensure that all skin barrier defence systems are in place, especially the acid mantle. Acids and enzymes are either keratolytic or proteolytic which means they will have some type of destructive effect upon the stratum corneum, therefore care must be taken with preparation of the skin and application of the solution.

As each of these modalities exhibit different properties, and ultimate choice would depend upon basic majority skin type and risk factors.
We now have a far greater understanding of the structure and function of the skin and the life cycle of the keratinocyte, and what we once believed to be a correct approach in the nineties would not be considered appropriate today. The chemistry we were taught is all still relevant, but we now approach skin differently, and with greater thought and respect for the skin barrier defence systems. Those immortal words *"Preserve the integrity of the epidermis at all times"* must always be remembered.

Alpha hydroxy acids

Most AHA's are used in formulations and clinical treatments because of their ability to help in the desquamation process, and for their antioxidant and hydrophilic properties.
AHA's are keratolytic, and this means that the chemical has the action of softening and loosening the desmosomes and physical bonds that hold the keratinocyte in place. Most AHA's are water soluble, with a small number water/oil soluble.
We will begin by putting acids into their respective categories. You will notice that each acid will have a slightly different action, and will therefore work better on some skin conditions and skin colours and not as well on others.

The pH is a major consideration to results

Before discussing different acids, we should review the relationship between the pH and the strength or percentage of acid in a formula, as it can be confusing to associate the two.
There is a percentage relationship connection with the pH level. Example: If you buy a glycolic acid at a 30% solution, then the pH value is most likely to be around 5 pH, and it would not be as effective as a glycolic acid at 10% with a pH value of 1.7. The lower pH value means the more effective the glycolic or acid of this type will be, and far more care with it's use will be required.
You will recall in chapter one where we initially discussed the pH scale, we discovered that it is logarithmic and a solution with a pH of 1.7 is actually over a thousand times more acidic than the 5 pH solution. This is why the pH 1.7 solution is far more diluted (%) than the pH 5.
The lowest and accepted pH was set by pharmaceutical regulatory bodies because it had been observed that unbuffered high percentage solutions has been applied to skins with disastrous results.

Glycolic acid (GA)

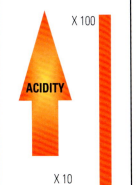

X 100

ACIDITY

X 10

pH 5   pH 4   pH 3

pH & Acidity Relationship

- Also known as hydroxyacetic acid, is synthetically manufactured for cosmetic use, but in nature it is derived from sugar cane and sugar beet and many other similar plant sources.
- Synthetic glycolic acid offers greater purity and quality (and more dependable consistency) than natural sources of glycolic acid and is effective in treating the condition of hyper-keratinisation due to its small molecular size.

- Because of this small molecular size and hygroscopic/hydrophilic qualities, it has the ability to realign the water phase of the lipid bilayers in the extracellular spaces of the stratum corneum.
- It is found in dermatological and skin treatment professional strength for clinical treatments, professional retail and domestic retail products.

Domestic use of GA

- In low concentrations, (2 - 5%) glycolic acid will facilitate progressive weakening of cohesion of the bilayers and corneo-desmosomes found in the stratum corneum (SC), assisting in uniform exfoliation of its outermost layers.
- At this low percentage it has been shown that no compromise of the skin barrier function of the skin occurs, and a more compact appearing SC is a result. These percentages are normally found in domestic retail products used for day care of facial and body skin.

Clinical use of GA

- Higher concentrations of glycolic acid used in the dermatological/professional skin treatments range from 30 to 70% with various pH's.
- The key to understanding how an acid can give the best result is not in the percentage of acid, nor is it in the "buffering".
- The key is in the pH of the acid; a lower pH will offer as good a result, if not better than a solution of 70% with a higher relative pH.

Best application of GA

- Glycolic acid is an excellent tool in the treatment of hyper-keratinisation for those skins that have accumulated years of neglect. Glycolic should not be the first choice if the skin is very lipid dry or the epidermis is compromised in some way.
- Always prepare a skin by rebuilding skin barrier defence systems first and this often takes about 3 weeks, then use an acid like glycolic to aid the desquamation of the keratinocyte.
- By preparing the skin, a deeper penetration of the acid will the result and the keratinocyte will be very responsive to the acid and its effects.
- A better realignment of the spinosum layer and a more complete and steady desquamation of the corneocyte will be the result of preparation combined with the action of the glycolic acid.

Blending glycolic with other acids & actives

- Recently there has been a revival of glycolic acid blended with fruit acids, there were a number of award winning blends in the mid nineties and these have once more found favour with therapist and their clients who wish a more subtle approach to this type of clinical resurfacing or treatment for hyper keratinisation.
- These are often referred to as glycolic/fruit acid cocktails and offer all of the action of glycolic acid plus the antioxidant action of the fruit acids.
- Glycolic blends well with many other types of actives for a wide range of skin conditions, with lactic acid, kojic acid and vitamin C a few of the most popular.

Take care

There will always be controversy about glycolic acid, and many clinicians unfortunately approach the use of acids without a second thought for the cells and systems of the epidermis and the long term ramifications of acids, or without other considerations of what the skin may require pre and post treatment.

Lactic acid

This acid is a carboxylic acid and has a molecular weight of 90.08. It is also known as 2-Hydroxypropanoic acid, or alpha-hydroxypropionic acid. The numbers C3H603 refer to its chemical number. It has a hydroxl group adjacent to the carboxyl group, making it an alpha hydroxy acid, and takes a number of forms:

- Lactic acid
- Sodium lactate
- Ammonium lactate

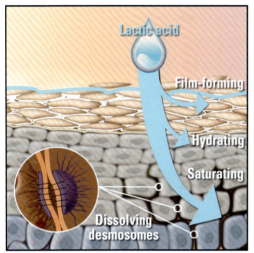

- Two major sources of lactic acid for cosmetic use are synthetic and fermented sugar (not milk). The fermented sugar form of lactic acid has shown to be very similar in form to the "free water of the epidermis" sometimes referred to as NMF or natural moisturising factor.
- Because of molecular weight and hydrophilic abilities, lactic acid is also known as a " film former". When it is applied to skin surface, it increases the stratum corneum extensibility and saturation/hydration capacity more than most other acids due to it's affinity to "free water" (NMF) of the epidermis.
- Consequently it has been found that lactic acid leaves more moisture behind than it takes from skin.

Suitable for compromised skins

Lactic acid for clinical use has many advantages and should be classified as a "first choice" for high-risk skins and photo types 3+ to 6.

If the skin is essential fatty acid deficient, has an impaired acid mantle or permanent diffused redness, peeling is not always the first choice treatments, however it could be introduced usually about 4 weeks into a treatment program.

Lactic acid will address resurfacing, hyper keratinisation and realignment of the bilayers of the epidermis without compromise of skin, and it's affinity and action with the ceramide content of the bilayers makes lactic acid an important component in the treatment of lipid dry skin.

Lactic acid as a tyrosinase inhibitor

- Lactic acid also has a mild tyrosinase inhibiting ability, making this acid a treatment choice in a skin-lightening program. Introduced at around 4 weeks into the preparation of the pigmented skin a number of results are achieved. The first is the psychological one, because skin immediately becomes clearer and brighter in appearance even after one treatment.

- The second is the tyrosinase inhibiting effect on the melanocyte, slowing down the formation of the pigment granules and contributing to the effectiveness of the chosen skin lightening products used at home and clinic.

- For hyper-keratinisation, lactic acid and other chemicals within that family have proven to be enormously successful, in addition lactic acid can be successfully blended with glycolic and other acids, and also used in combination with resorcinol and salicylic acid to become the Jessner's peel.

Ammonium lactate

- Ammonium lactate is a combination of neutralised lactic acid and ammonium hydroxide, and in 12% emulsions has been shown to relieve symptoms of dry skin. Frequent use shows a significant reduction in hyper-keratinisation, dryness and TEWL.
- Topical ammonium lactate produces a remission in people suffering from skin disorders such as ichthyosis, psoriasis and keratosis pilaris.

Mandelic acid

- Also known as alpha-hydroxybenzeneacetic acid, this acid and its many derivatives are used for their dual activities as an antibacterial agent and for assisting in desquamation of the keratinocyte by the dissolution of desmosomes.
- This property makes it a suitable chemical for the treatment of non inflammatory grades acne 1 & 2 (open and closed comedones) and inflammatory acne grade 3 (10 pustules or less).
- The larger molecular size may also be a reason why mandelic shows fewer negative side effects with use, the size would slow penetration therefore keeping the chemical at the surface where it would have a saturating effect similar to lactic acid.

Fruit Acids

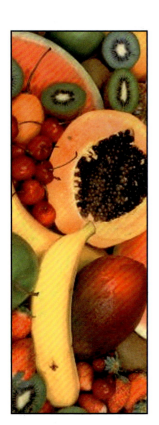

Fruit acids are very widely used in the cosmetic industry, as antioxidant, preservative, acid and alkali buffers and also tyrosinase inhibitors. Technically, fruit acids are not AHA's but for simpler marketing purposes they were placed under the same banner.

Citric acid would be one of the most widely used fruit acids, and although citric acid has origins in the citrus world of fruits, most citric acid used in cosmetics are synthetic. Clients who wish their cosmetics to have a "natural" image will gravitate toward cosmetics that contain "fruit anything".

Citric acid

- Citric acid is an alpha hydroxy acid that can be extracted from citrus fruits or made from fermented sugar solutions. Lemon juice contains 5 to 8% citric acid. Calcium citrate, potassium citrate and sodium citrate are salts of citric acid.
- In cosmetics and personal care products, citric acid and its calcium, potassium and sodium salts may function as chelating agents, or pH adjusters. The salts may also function as buffering agents, and citric acid may function as a fragrance ingredient.

Malic acid

- Malic acid is an intermediate in the Krebs cycle of a cell, (as is citric acid) and in the instances of skin the keratinocyte would be the cell that should come to mind.
- Malic acid is a colourless, crystalline aliphatic dicarboxylic acid that occurs naturally in a wide variety of unripe fruit and is commonly used as a pH alkali buffer in cosmetics.
- Sodium malate is the sodium salt of malic acid.

Tartaric acid

- Tartaric acid is an organic carboxylic acid salt. It occurs naturally in many plants, particularly grapes and tamarinds. Salts of tartaric acid are called tartrates. These salts include calcium tartrate, potassium tartrate, potassium sodium tartrate and disodium tartrate.
- Tartaric acid and its salts are used as pH adjusters in cosmetics and personal care products.

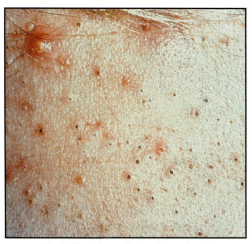

Oil solubility makes salicylic acid a preferred choice for skins with open comedones.

Beta hydroxy acids

A simple comparison between beta hydroxy acids (BHA's) and alpha hydroxy acids (AHA's) is that BHA's are primarily oil soluble and therefore have affinity with the oil phases of the bilayers and sebaceous gland secretions. Conversely, AHA's are water-soluble and have a great affinity with the water phase of the bilayers of the stratum corneum and other water-soluble epidermal structures.

Salicylic acid

Salicylic acid is classified as a BHA and can be obtained from the bark of willow trees. Salicylic acid and its salts and esters have many functions; these ingredients may be used in many types of cosmetics and personal care products, from wart remover to fragrance enhancer to UV light absorber to solvent. Caution should be taken when using this acid in high concentrations on darker skins, (Photo types 4 to 6) as post inflammatory pigmentation can occur under certain circumstances.

The salts of salicylic acid are:

- Calcium salicylate
- Potassium salicylate
- Magnesium salicylate
- Sodium salicylate
- MEA-Salicylate
- TEA-Salicylate

The esters of salicylic acid are:

- Butyloctyl salicylate
- Hexyldecyl salicylate
- Ethylhexyl salicylate
- Tridecyl salicylate
- C12-15 Alkyl salicylate
- Isocetyl salicylate
- Methyl salicylate
- Capryolyl salicylic acid
- Isodecyl salicylate
- Myristyl salicylate

Clinical treatment with salicylic acid

- For the treatment of skin conditions related to hyper-keratinisation, salicylic acid has great strength in the treatment of chronic oily skin, non-inflammatory acne grade 2 (open comedones) and inflammatory acne grade 3.
- The reason for this is the oil solubility of the acid, allowing faster and more efficient access down the oil gland in addition having access to the epidermal layers as well.
- It has been suggested that lower percentages of salicylic acid can produce better results than higher percentages of an AHA.
- It would be my suggestion that a clinician should carry BHA's and a selection of AHA's for clinical treatments to offer the best to their clients.

ßeta-lipohydroxy acid (C8-Lipohydroxy acid) (LHA)

- This salicylic acid derivative with lipophilic abilities provides slow penetration into skin, with this slower diffusion generally resulting in less of an inflammatory response and reduced redness after treatment. This makes it suitable for oily skins with open comedones and inflammatory acne grade 3.
- In addition to it's keratolytic properties, this acid helps decrease bacterial concentration inside the pilo-sebaceous duct by impairing attachment of the bacteria to the cellular debris within.

Other desquamating acids

Trichloroacetic acid (TCA)

- TCA is a synthetic chemical based on acetic acid. In order to make the acid more active, three chloride atoms are substituted for three hydrogen atoms. TCA is available to trained skin treatment therapists in low concentrations of 0.5% to 10%. It has been developed with a built-in control factor that works by stopping its action when the solution dries on the skin surface.

- These new TCA's offer a more comfortable treatment for the client, (heat versus prickling sensation) and a weak dilution of the solution will offer better results than the once favoured higher percentages of glycolic peels. It is however, a strong acid and significantly deep destruction of the skin can be produced if not using recognised brands or without appropriate training.

- TCA peels are only suitable for Photo type 1 to 3, and care should be taken to ascertaining the skins "risk factor" for pigmentation, scarring and marking. The reason for this caution is we can no longer rely on the older method of phototyping a skin due to the diverse cross-ethnic characteristics of modern society.

Jessner's peel

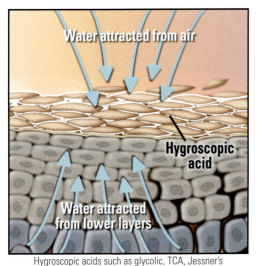

Hygroscopic acids such as glycolic, TCA, Jessner's and phenol peels all attract water from surrounding tissue and atmosphere. Preparation of the skin and adequate epidermal hydration levels are therefore vital to treatment success.

- The basic formulation of the Jessner's peel consists of a mixture or lactic, salicylic and resorcinol in equal amounts in an ethanol solution. Various modifications such as lowering the amount of resorcinol reduces the toxicity of this formula, and reduces " down time" or recovery period at the expense of peeling results.
- The depth of peel achieved is dependant on the number of layers applied, and even experienced clinicians would not apply more than seven layers. The pattern of application is very important, as is the preparation of the skin before treatment. This peel is not for those skins that are compromised or unprepared, and this means that a number of preparatory clinical treatments before the peel is advisable.
- Post care is a little different to other types of peels, in that the skin should not be washed or cleansed until the peeling action has completed and this may be as long as seven days. (Depending on the number of layers applied and depth of peel).

Phenol peels (Carbolic acid)

- Phenol peels (Carbolic acid) have been in use since the 1970's and are still in use from quite strong to lighter special solutions. They are the deepest type of peel and use the strongest chemical solutions.
- It is contraindicated for photo types 3 to 6, and unsuitable for the neck area. Disadvantages include the potential to cause permanent skin lightening by reducing the skin's ability to produce pigment, and the requirement for increased sun protection (Post treatment) for life.
- Laser resurfacing has largely replaced these peels as the modality of choice for those who wish to treat deep wrinkles and scarring.
- In lighter solutions it is very effective in preparing skin for extractions, and is being added to cleansers in very weak solutions to aid the desquamation process of congested skin.

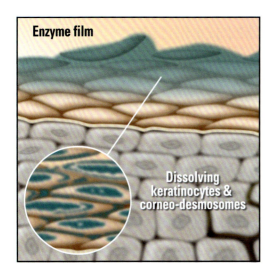

Enzyme film

Dissolving
keratinocytes &
corneo-desmosomes

Enzymes

Enzyme therapy is a growing and widely respected modality in the treatment of many skin conditions, with the skin treatment industry using enzymes as an effective treatment modality for hyper-keratinisation and related skin conditions of non inflammatory grade acne 1 & 2 and inflammatory grade acne 3.

Enzymes are proteolytic, and this means that the chemical will dissolve or digest proteins. Since the keratinocyte and corneocyte are proteins of keratin, the complete cell including the desmosomes and bonds that hold it in place are digested.

For an enzyme to be activated there will always need to be a catalyst available and in the case of most treatments, this is water.

Some treatments however, supply a special catalyst solution.

Bromelain or Papaine

- The enzymes papaine and bromelain historically used in clinical treatments were derived from papaya and pineapple, although more modern formulas use synthetics.
- Used in masks and peeling solutions, this type of treatment offers an immediate solution because the skin cell is digested immediately. There is generally no eight-day waiting period for desquamation as is the case when using AHA's.

Peptides for hyper-keratinisation

The cell adhesion proteins of the desmosome are called the desmoglein and desmocollin. They are proteins that bridge the space between epithelial cells such as the keratinocyte.

We have learnt that to have efficient desquamation of a corneocyte the desmosomes must be completely dissolved by hydophilic enzymes. Up until recently AHA's and enzymes or physical actions such as micro-dermabrasion have been the only methods that would assist in desquamation of the corneocyte in the treatment of hyper-keratinisation, however there are now peptides available for this treatment.

Biomimetic peptides

- This new peptide technology has meant another methodology of treatment of this skin condition is now available. Peptides that were similar to the cell adhesion recognition sites of desmoglein were found to specifically prevent desmosome adhesion. As these peptides reduce the corneocyte cell-to-cell adhesion, they effectively contribute to better desquamation.

- A new active cosmetic ingredient known as Perfection-Peptide P3, contains the tripeptide with the amino acid residue sequence of the cell adhesion recognition sites of desmoglein.
- The precise chemical structure of the peptide is hexanoyl-Arg-Ala-Nle-NH2.
- The length of the peptide was restricted to the cell adhesion recognition site in order to ensure penetration of the peptide into the deeper stratum corneum, (Peptide size often limits penetration) and to further aid diffusion, encapsulated in lecithin liposomes.

certain chemicals and move to the source of these "chemo-attractants" or "smell". The chemotaxis (change of behaviour according to chemical environment) by P. acnes lipase indicated a wider role for this enzyme in the inflammatory process and the development of acne vulgaris.

Benzoyl peroxide

- Benzoyl peroxide (BP) is used as an antibacterial ingredient that has the ability to indirectly reduce the free fatty acids that are involved in the inflammatory response of acne. It is the peroxide action of BP that causes an oxidative situation within the pilosebaceous duct where it is theorised that free radicals are generated in the process of reducing the P. acnes population.

- A potentially more negative side of benzoyl peroxide is that it can cause post inflammatory pigmentation on skins phototype 4 and higher. This means that it is unsuitable for skins of "high risk". Benzoyl peroxide has a known photo sensitising effect, and because of this should not be worn in the sun, and if used, only applied at night. Ensure that it is completely removed in the morning by using a cleanser and toner followed by an antioxidant gel and sun protection.

Note: In 1995, the FDA changed benzoyl peroxide to a Category III (safety is unknown) status, and even though there have been numerous studies associating its long term use with the development of carcinomas, it still remains available without prescription globally.

Hyper-keratinisation, comedones & inflammatory acne #3 : Chemical treatment solutions

Product characteristics & suitability	Compromised skin	High risk skin	Keratolytic	Proteolytic	Oil soluble	Water soluble	Saturating	Hydrating	Hygroscopic	Anti-bacterial	Antioxidant	5a-reductase inhibitor	Tyrosinase inhibitor	Peptides
Glycolic acid	✓	✓	✓			✓			✓					
Lactic acid	✓	✓	✓			✓	✓	✓			✓		✓	
Salicylic acid			✓	✓						✓				
Mandelic acid	✓	✓	✓			✓	✓	✓		✓				
Fruit acids	✓	✓	✓			✓	✓	✓		✓	✓			
Biomimetic peptides	✓	✓	✓		✓	✓		✓						✓
Papaine	✓	✓		✓		✓		✓		✓	✓			
Bromelaine	✓	✓		✓		✓		✓		✓	✓			
Jessner's peel			✓			✓	✓	✓						
TCA peel			✓			✓				✓				
Phenol peel			✓			✓				✓				
Azealic acid	✓	✓	✓			✓				✓	✓	✓	✓	
Vitamin B3	✓	✓				✓					✓	✓		
Tea tree oil				✓						✓	✓			
Benzoyl peroxide			✓							✓				
Vitamin B6	✓	✓				✓		✓		✓	✓			
Zinc	✓	✓								✓	✓			

Skin condition: Loss of structural integrity & thin skin density

Collagen's loss of structural integrity is also a condition related to texture, and we will briefly review the cells & systems of concern involved in this skin condition so we can relate it to product composition more easily. A full anatomy & physiology of these cells and systems will be found in the advanced skin analysis book pages 34-47.

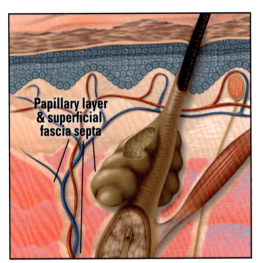

Papillary layer & superficial fascia septa

The superficial fascia septa (a sheath of loose connective tissue) surrounds all appendages and structures within the dermis.

Connective tissue

Collagen is the principle protein constituent of the fibrous connective tissues. It is part of the weave of the skin, its principle function being to help maintain the resistance, strength and structural integrity in the tissues.

Fibroblasts are responsible for making collagen, elastin and glycosaminoglycans, and have abundant rough endoplasmic reticulum and well-developed golgi to make these specialised proteins. Normal repair and replacement of collagen and elastin proteins will see minor activity of the fibroblast.

To obtain full activity and division of this cell and increased growth factors, the wound-healing processes would have to be stimulated.

Ageing processes will follow the superficial fascia pathway

The papillary layer and rete pegs are the first areas of the dermis to age, and this ageing process will follow the superficial fascia septa that surrounds and supports all appendages (E.G. capillaries and sebaceous glands) in the dermis. This sheath then continues down through reticular and subcutaneous layers in a vertical manner until reaching the muscle and deep fascia septa.

Understanding the vertical progression of ageing down through the superficial fascia septa is key to choosing appropriate modalities and writing a treatment pathway. In addition to tissue deterioration, there will be an associated ageing of the fibroblasts or cellular damage, and the deeper down this vertical path into the fascia septa the damage, the more radical the solution required. These factors will dictate modality and treatment choice, and how successful any treatment will be.

Fibroblast requirements to make collagen

A cell will only produce what it is programmed to create, and this is providing it's nutritional requirements such as amino acids and enzymes to stimulate cell production are met. Knowing the basics of the fibroblast's requirement is key to choosing the right product composition as it has a very comprehensive list of necessary things to make collagen, elastin and glycosaminoglycans. They are as follows:

- Vitamin C
- Growth factors and hormones
- Iron (Co factor)
- Silicon allied with magnesium and calcium
- EFA's for cellular function & healthy cell membranes

- Bioflavonoids
- Zinc (Co factor)
- Key Amino acids (proline & lysine)

- Vitamin A
- Copper peptides

From these vitamins, minerals, hormones and growth factors, a selection of treatment and product actives can be found. Many have already been discussed in a previous chapter, and this discussion will refer back to that chapter, and also revisit some again but from a different perspective.

Fibroblast nutrition

Of course, it is obvious that some of these elements can only be obtained through nutritional sources and would never be viable in a cosmetic formulation.

Therefore, supplements to assist in skin metabolism and health are recommended as part of the home care program.

Treatment solutions for loss of structural integrity & thin skin density

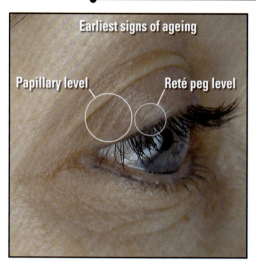

Earliest signs of ageing

Papillary level   Reté peg level

Small vertical lines along the lashes indicate collagen deterioration and flattening of reté pegs. This is one of the early signs of ageing. The longer vertical lines indicate the level of collagen deterioration to be progressing further down through the papillary layer.

Note: Only those actives that have a proven history of success will be discussed in this section. Not covered are actives that are considered alternative or still under review.

Choosing the right treatment actives

This is the next part of cosmetic chemistry that the clinician must learn, and the choices made for an ageing skin are based on the protocols of skin type and skin colour. This improves the chances and success rate of the treatment regime. Ageing skin with loss of structural integrity will normally exhibit the following levels of cellular damage and tissue changes:

- Lipid dry
- Diffused redness
- Lipid peroxidation
- Mitochondria DNA damage to keratinocyte, and fibroblast
- Cellular senescence of the melanocyte (around 15% of cells)
- Fascia septa deterioration at upper reticular level (at minimum)

What can be established from these levels of tissue and cellular damage is that the oil phases of the skin barrier defence systems as well as cell membranes have all been compromised. This is in addition to the deterioration the connective tissue collagen. The treatment methodologies best suited for remedial intervention should repair, replace and maintain those lipid phases and be able to stimulate collagen deposition without compromising the protocols of diffused redness and thin skin density.

Vitamin C as a co-factor in collagen synthesis

Ascorbic acid is required by the body to produce collagen - the fibrous structural protein of connective tissues. It is the matrix on which bones and teeth are formed, and the triple helix that "holds" dermal tissue together, and re-connects separated tissues forming scars.

Beyond its function in collagen formation, ascorbic acid is known to increase absorption of inorganic iron, to have essential roles in the metabolism of folic acid and of some amino acids and hormones, and to act as an antioxidant.

Collagen protein requires vitamin C and iron for "hydroxylation" - the addition of an OH group - or the conversion of the amino acids proline and lysine to hydroxyproline and hydroxylysine.

These substances facilitate the binding together of collagen fibres into strong "rope-like" triple helix structures. Without vitamin C and iron, hydroxylation does not take place, and collagen fails to produce triple helixes resulting in weak connective tissues. This may interfere with wound healing and accelerate the ageing process.

Ascorbic acid

In chapter one, all forms of vitamin C were covered in depth. (pages 64 to 70) The variations in the benefits and blends of each type of ascorbic acid means that not all are suitable for an ageing skin, and there will be some that would be chosen in preference to another.

Reference points of base line ascorbic acid

- Water-soluble.
- Antioxidant.
- Acidic & slightly desquamating (compromised skin will need to acclimatise).
- Combines well with other skin vitamins and co enzymes.
- Encapsulated L-ascorbic acid will mean reduced acidity and more suitable for a mature ageing skin, however skin still may take time to acclimatise due to reduced skin lipid levels.

The key points benefits and clinical use of each recommended type of ascorbic acid are listed here.

Magnesium ascorbyl phosphate (MAP or VWMg) for collagen synthesis

- Less acidic than ascorbic acid.
- Very suitable for compromised skins. (No need to acclimatise)
- Suitable for aged skin.
- Very suitable for skin that exhibit "high risk" for pigmentation.
- Combined with magnesium and phosphate (two more very essential elements for collagen synthesis) giving greater access of ascorbic acid to the cell interior.
- Lower concentrations (compared to ascorbic acid) are required to deliver the same amount of ascorbic acid into the cell.
- Longer shelf life.

Ascorbyl tetraisopalmitate: an oil soluble form of Vitamin C for collagen synthesis

- This type of vitamin C is rendered oil soluble with the addition of four palmitic acid ions.
- It is lipophilic, and easily penetrates the stratum corneum bilayers.
- Lipid solubility means that up to ten times more vitamin C absorption than water soluble version.
- Lipid solubility means more effective control of melanin formation.
- More efficient protection against oxidative stress and lipid peroxidation.
- Very suitable for lipid dry compromised skin.
- Extremely stable in formulations, does not oxidize easily, providing longer shelf life.

Vitamin C ester for collagen synthesis

- Vitamin C esters ascorbyl palmitate, or ascorbyl di-palmitate, are still effective at transferring through the lipid bi-layers and getting through into the cell.
- Esters as a cosmetic ingredient, they can be natural or synthetic and liquid or solid depending on properties of the reacting substances.
- Being insoluble in water, they replace oils and fats to provide uniform composition and preservation, they have good skin tolerance and a lubricating and emollient action.

Vitamin C summary

You will see from these choices of vitamin C that they are either oil soluble, (and able to care for the cell membrane, reduce oxidative stress and lipid peroxidation) or have been combined with other elements that the cell requires and has receptors for.
This latter feature ensures better assimilation into the cell interior. These points will all lead towards quicker collagen synthesis and firmer, denser connective tissue of the papillary layer and the superficial fascia septa.

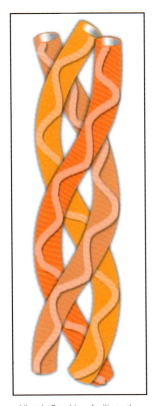

Vitamin C and iron facilitate the binding together of collagen fibres in to strong "rope like" triple helix structures.

Key amino acids: proline and lysine

- The amino acids proline and lysine are metabolised by vitamin C, both of these amino acids are key in the manufacture of collagen type 1 & 3.
- Lysyl hydroxylase and prolyl hydroxylase enzymes of the proline & lysine amino acids are essential for collagen synthesis.
- High levels of essential amino acids, enzymes and B group vitamins have many different sources, as cosmetic ingredient actives, the most common and acceptably used is the marine source of amino acids such as seaweed and the fresh water algae spirulina.
- The amino acid proline exhibits antioxidant abilities and works well with super dismutase oxide in formulations.

Bioflavonoids for collagen synthesis

Bioflavonoids are antioxidants that work with and care for other antioxidants to offer a complete system of protection. Numerous studies have shown bioflavonoids unique role in protecting vitamin C from oxidation in the body, thereby allowing the body to reap more benefits from vitamin C.
Note that all three of the listed bioflavonoids have an additional effect on the circulatory system, making them a positive in a formulation for any product linked to the skin conditions known as loss of structural integrity and thin skin density which is the ageing skin.

Pycnogenol™

- Active ingredient is proanthocyanidin. (OPC)
- History of success in treating vascular conditions, reducing inflammation and slowing angiogenesis of the capillary network. Because diffused redness is behind and part of the thin skin density of an aging skin, it is a good choice.

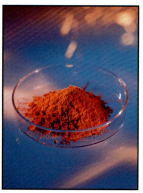

Pycnogenol™ is the brand name for an extract made from the Maritime pine tree.

Grape seed extract (Vitis vinefera)

- Contains proanthocyanidin, and so this extract has the same beneficial effects on the circulatory system as Pycnogenol™.
- Inhibits blood platelet aggregation and reduces inflammation. (Anti-inflammatory)
- Good support for lessening oxidative stress and the resulting lipid peroxidation that follows.

Green tea extract (Camellia sinensis)

- Ability to inhibit the MMP enzyme collagenase. This is vitally important when treating an aged or frequently sun exposed skin.
- The methylxanthines content of green tea works on the small capillaries of the microcirculation reducing angiogenesis, as do the flavonoids and catechols reducing erythema.
- Some research has shown that green tea exhibits a photo protective effect and is now being formulated into sun protection products.

Vitamin A for collagen synthesis

Reference points of base line vitamin A

- Lipophilic
- Oil soluble
- Antioxidant
- Non-inflammatory
- Reduces oxidative stress
- Reduces lipid peroxidation
- Re-activates vitamin A receptors
- High percentage naturally found in the epidermis
- Restores cellular homeostasis

The key points benefits and clinical use of each recommended type of vitamin A.

Retinyl palmitate & ßeta carotene for collagen synthesis

- 80% of the vitamin A naturally found in the skin is in the form of retinyl palmitate.
- Vitamin A esters, retinyl palmitate and beta-carotene are less irritating to the skin.
- Studies show that same results will be achieved as using more aggressive versions of vitamin A.
- The esters of vitamin A play a pivotal role in cell metabolism and homeostasis.
- Vitamin A cellular receptors numbers are increased by the topical application of retinyl palmitate.
- Retinyl palmitate is converted into retinol as it passes through the cell membrane.
- Retinol is converted to retinoic acid within the cell, increasing DNA activity.
- Oil solubility makes this ester ideal for the treatment of oxidative stress and lipid peroxidation.

ßeta carotene

- Another ester of vitamin A is ßeta-carotene and this is normally found throughout the epidermis.
- ßeta carotene has well known antioxidant properties and can neutralize many free radicals.
- The oil solubility of makes this ester another ideal prevention and treatment of oxidative stress and lipid peroxidation.
- Works well with sun protection formulations.

Retinol for collagen synthesis

- Retinol is the alcohol form of vitamin A and may be more irritating if the skin has not been acclimatised, or has limited numbers of vitamin A receptors in the cell membrane.
- Passes quickly through the epidermis to cell producing layers such as the basal layer, then hydrolyses into retinyl palmitate so as to be compatible with the cell receptor.
- Retinol is converted to retinoic acid once inside the cell (intracellular)
- Retinol actively encourages mitochondria formation of retinoic acid for DNA and cellular division
- Storage and shelf life need care and attention (check packaging)

Florence says: It is from a cellular point that these forms of vitamin A are preferable for the ageing skin with thin skin density. The oil solubility of the esters of vitamin A accessibility through the epidermis is easy (via skin lipids). Having receptors for retinyl palmitate also means quick access to the cell interior and the mitochondria, which is where all the action takes place.
Vitamin A is one of our biggest weapons against ageing alongside peptides and growth factors.

Vitamin A

Vitamin A in the form of retinyl palmitate is measured in international units (IU) per gram. When expressed as a percentage in a solution, 10,000 IU/ g is the equivelant of 1% per gram.

As an example:
7,000 IU/ g = 0.7% per g and
2,500 IU/ g = 0.25% per g

The recommended effective doses of topical application are between 500 IU and 10, 000 IU per application.

Anything less than 500 IU (Or 0.2% per g) is generally of no therapeutic value and is less than what would be in a cream for diaper rash.

Peptides for collagen synthesis

Copper peptides

Copper is one of the elements that the fibroblast requires for collagen synthesis; therefore this peptide fits into that role very well. Certain kinds of peptides have an avid affinity for copper, to which they bind very tightly. The resulting compound consisting of a peptide and a copper atom has become known as a copper peptide. The mechanism of copper peptide action is relatively complex. The peptide chain of glycyl-L-histidyl-L-lysine-Cu (GHK-Cu) promotes the synthesis of elastin, proteoglycans, glycosaminoglycans and other components of the dermis and has been found to work very well in the early phases of wound healing by encouraging the placement of wound collagen, in addition it has shown to improve older connective tissue found in scars.

The ability to regulate the growth rate and migration of different types of cells; significant anti-inflammatory action; and the ability to prevent the release of oxidation-promoting iron into the tissues. The net result is a faster, better and "cleaner" healing.

Other peptides that target collagen synthesis

- Palmitoyl oligopeptide
- Palmitoyl tetrapeptide 7
- Matrixyl 3000®
- Kinetin

All of these peptides have research history of influencing collagen deposition, particularly the palmitoyl oligopeptide and Matrixyl®. I refer you back to pages 32 and 33 in the first chapter to refresh yourself with the amino acids that are used to make these peptides and their affinity to collagen synthesis.

Designer peptides

Formulators are creating custom anti-aging peptides such as Matrixyl 3000® and Oligopeptides from amino acids.

Growth factors for collagen synthesis

Growth factors are compounds that act as chemical messengers between cells; regulating a variety of cellular activities. To date, all growth factors used by the cosmetic industry are from bovine sources in the form of colostrum polypeptides. Bovine colostrum contains insulin, and transforming growth factors. In some exclusive anti-ageing clinics, their growth factors are supplied from a controversial variety of sources including cultured epidermal cells, placental cells, colostrum, human foreskin and even plants.

Macrophage derived growth factors are naturally stimulated during wound healing, and clinicians that are practising the medical needling modality or recommending the client use the 0.2mm or 0.5mm roller for home use would be very knowledgeable about the advantages of stimulating growth factors for the treatment of an ageing skin.

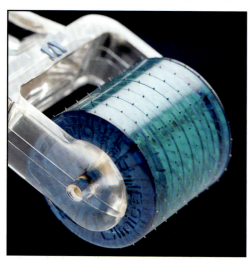

- Growth factors are required for any stage of collagen replacement or repair and some form of modality that would simulate a wound healing response should ideally be part of the process.
- Growth factors have been used extensively in the medical industry for treating wounds to facilitate faster and more complete healing.
- Growth factors play a role in cell division, new cell and blood vessel growth, including collagen and elastin production and distribution.

Supporting fluids of the dermis (Glycosaminoglycans GAGs)

Glycosaminoglycans (GAGs), is the major fluid of the dermis formed by the fibroblast. It is this fluid that plays the important role of creating what we call the "dermal reserve" by surrounding and supporting collagen and elastin fibrils.
A major component of GAGs (around 70%) is hyaluronic acid (HA), a large hydrophilic polysaccharide consisting of glucuronic acid and glucosamine that attracts water. When tissues are undergoing growth or repair, levels of GAGs increases.
The GAGs draw plasma containing oxygen and nutrients from the microcirculatory system to form the blend known as the " dermal reserve". It is this fluid that supply dermal cells such as the fibroblast with the nutrients required for cellular function. It will further seep through the sinusoidal connective tissue of the dermal/epidermal junction to also supply the cells of the epidermis with nutrients and oxygen.

Hyaluronic acid (HA) Sodium hyaluronate as a supporting dermal reserve fluid

- Hyaluronic acid has a high molecular weight and is very hydrophilic. It functions as a 'molecular sponge" allowing extensive hydration.
- HA can also function as a transdermal delivery system for other "actives" since it forms a matrix on the skin, allowing increased skin penetration due to saturation and hydration of tissue.
- Because of the unique hydrophilic abilities and molecular weight of hyaluronic acid it can be classified as a "giving humectant". This means that in addition to attracting water it is "film forming" and this is a very attractive result for a cosmetic ingredient.
- The hyaluronic acid used in products has varying sources. Some come from a sterile, bio-fermentation extraction process, which is labelled "synthetic." Other sources of hyaluronic acid, which are often labelled "natural," may include rooster-comb and bovine ocular-material.

Glucosamine as a supporting dermal reserve fluid

- Glucosamine is the building block for larger molecules such as hyaluronic acid, which is a major component of the connective tissue (dermal reserve).
- Hyaluronic acid (HA) levels decline with age and it is believed that by increasing the levels of glucosamine will increase the production of HA, improving the support for collagen and elastin.
- There is the added synergy of using glucosamine with niacinamide (B3) for the treatment of ageing skin. Niacinamide slows down the transfer of the melanin granule to the keratinocyte and glucosamine also interferes with the formation of tyrosinase in addition to being a precursor to hyaluronic acid. Together they offer a reduction in the formation of melanin in the epidermis and an increase in the supporting connective tissue of the dermis.

Chitin as a supporting dermal reserve fluid

- Chitin, the main constituent of the crustacean shells, is an excellent cosmetic product that is remarkably well tolerated by the skin.
- Chitin works like hyaluronic acid and increases the hydration levels of the epidermis.
- The chemical structure of chitin, a natural polymer, is very close to that of glycosaminoglycans (heparin and hyaluronic acid), whose biological tolerance has been demonstrated for a long time.
- Chitin is an efficient trapper of heavy metals that are responsible for very many contact allergies; therefore it is great for inflammatory response.

Glucosamine supplements

Synovial fluid of joints is also made by the fibroblast, and although similar to the glycosaminoglycans of the dermis, there are some subtle differences, such as the presence of chondroitin sulphate.
Client joint discomfort or pain can be an indicating diagnostic tool in ascertaining if there is a decline in the level of glycosaminoglycans being made by the fibroblast. This reflects that possibly there will be a reduction in the level of supporting fluids of the dermis and this will manifest as an accelerated ageing process. Glucosamine supplements should be recommended as part of the home care program for ageing skin.

DMAE for an ageing skin (Dimethylaminoethanol)

As you have read there are many types of antioxidants that should be a basic part of skins daily regime, there are some that are especially great for loss of structural integrity, oxidative stress and lipid peroxidation. In addition to showing excellent results as an antioxidant, DMAE also has proven to have additional benefits.

- Active anti-inflammatory effect making it suitable for compromised thin skin with diffused redness.
- The modulating effect on epidermal cells means a better cell-to-cell adhesion of desmosomes, improved density of spinosum layer that reflects into a more even placement of pigment by the melanocyte.
- The innate immune system is also strengthened because of better cellular memory of the keratinocyte, and the epidermal environment is functioning with more efficient langerhans cells.

DMAE in conjunction with the antioxidants vitamin C and lipoic acid makes for a wonderful anti-ageing cocktail of ingredients. Read more about DMAE in the segment on pigmentation.

Zinc a co-factor in collagen synthesis

- Zinc is required for collagen production and elastin synthesis.
- It is required for DNA repair and for DNA duplication, which is required for cell division.
- It is required for the production of superoxide dismutase, a powerful skin antioxidant.
- Zinc is a co-factor in the skin's production of certain metalloproteinases (MMP's) that remove damaged tissue.

Calcium for the ageing skin

One of the major concerns with an aging skin is the reduction in the density and thickness of the spinosum layer and the loss of the connection of the epidermis to the dermal epidermal junction. When these layer become separated the result can be visually devastating and compound all aspects of an ageing skin, therefore one of the treatment pathways is to keep the keratinocytes keratin content strong to ensure strong even connection is maintained by hemi-desomosmes and desmosomes.

- Calcium regulates keratinocyte differentiation, therefore having a greater effect on the epidermis and keratin fibril strength.
- One of the keratinocytes cells last functions before desquamation is to trigger the production of an enzyme named "protein kinase C", this enzyme is stimulated by the calcium content of the keratinocyte.
- The enzyme protein kinase C will travel back to basal cell layer to stimulate the immature keratinocyte to begin the keratinisation and differentiation process.
- High levels of calcium will mean faster rapid cell turnover and stronger keratin fibril and corneocytes of the stratum corneum.
- It has also been found that absorbable topical calcium has a beneficial effect on the bilayers of the stratum corneum, assisting in the formation of this important skin barrier defence system.
- Calcium assists in the formation of the first three lines of skin barrier defence

A lower level of calcium is typical of the ageing skin and this can reflect in other ways apart from thin skin density and being fragile, easy to mark and bruise, for example osteoporosis. Watch for these indications during the consultation process.

Summary

There are perhaps a number of anti-ageing actives that have not been mentioned in this section, and with the large number of these ingredients available, (and growing) it is not possible to list them all. The goal with this segment was to target the cellular requirements of the fibroblast to make collagen, elastin and glycosaminoglycans. What has to be realised that these actives mentioned are the **basic actives** that an anti-ageing skin care line and treatment regime should possess.

At absolute **minimum**, three of these components should be present in some form. The more of these in a daily regime, the more effective the results.

Omega's have not been mentioned in this section (Even though critical to an cellular heath) as they are mentioned later in this book in the more appropriate secretions section.

Product characteristics & suitability	Compromised skin	High risk skin	Collagen synthesis	Glycosaminoglycans	Oxidative stress	Lipid peroxidation	Antioxidant	Anti-inflammatory	Oil soluble	Tyrosinase inhibitor	Peptides	Acidic	Shelf life	Stability
Ascorbic acid	✓	✓	✓	✓	✓		✓	✓		✓		✓		
Magnesium ascorbyl phosphate	✓	✓	✓	✓	✓		✓	✓		✓			✓	
Ascorbyl tetra isopalmitate	✓	✓	✓	✓	✓	✓	✓	✓	✓	✓			✓	✓
Ascorbic esters	✓	✓	✓	✓	✓	✓	✓	✓	✓	✓			✓	
Bioflavonoids	✓	✓					✓	✓		✓				
Amino acid proline	✓	✓	✓	✓			✓	✓					✓	✓
Amino acid lysine	✓	✓	✓	✓			✓	✓					✓	✓
ßeta carotene	✓	✓			✓	✓	✓	✓	✓				✓	✓
Retinyl palmitate	✓	✓	✓		✓	✓	✓	✓	✓				✓	✓
Retinol			✓	✓			✓	✓						
Copper peptide	✓	✓	✓	✓			✓	✓		✓	✓		✓	✓
Matrixyl®	✓	✓	✓	✓			✓	✓		✓	✓		✓	✓
Growth factors	✓	✓	✓	✓	✓		✓	✓						
Hyaluronic acid	✓	✓	✓	✓	✓	✓	✓	✓		✓			✓	✓
Glucosamine	✓	✓	✓	✓	✓	✓	✓	✓		✓			✓	✓
Chitin	✓	✓	✓	✓			✓	✓					✓	✓
Calcium	✓	✓	✓	✓	✓	✓	✓	✓					✓	✓
DMAE	✓	✓	✓	✓	✓	✓	✓	✓		✓			✓	✓
Zinc	✓	✓	✓	✓	✓	✓	✓	✓					✓	✓

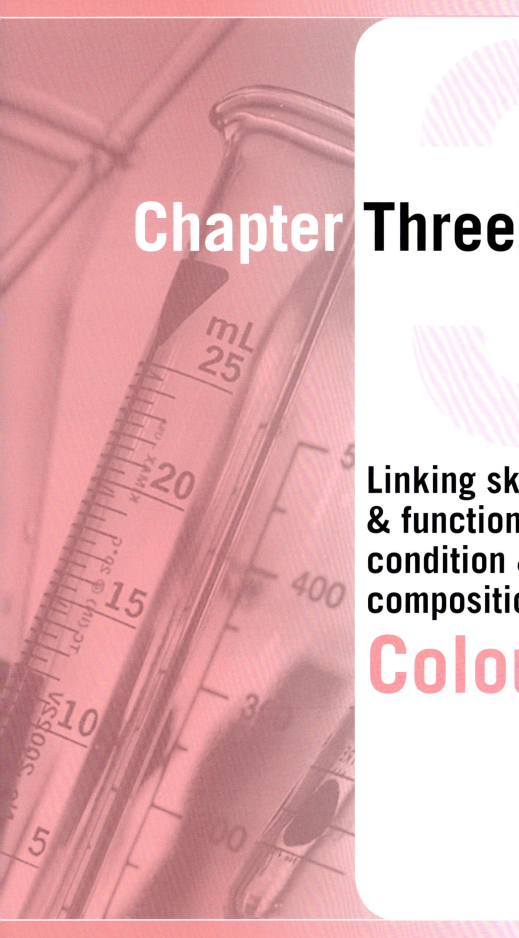

Chapter Three

Linking skin structure & function to skin condition & product composition

Colour

Skin conditions that alter the colour of skin

As with skin texture, there are a number of factors that control the colour of the skin. Some of these factors are external, (That influence the epidermis) and some are internal (That influence the dermis). Again, we will examine these two categories of cells and systems separately to help make them easier to remember and understand.

Epidermal

Pigmentation plays a major role in the colour of the skin, and conditions related to the abnormal production of melanin (hyper-pigmentation and hypo-pigmentation) are not uncommon.
By understanding melanogenesis (formation of melanin pigment granules) the melanocyte life cycle, and how it works in synergy with the keratinocyte, you will be able to ascertain the cause of pigmented skin conditions and put in place an effective treatment program.

Dermal

The microcirculation plays a very large role in the overall colour of the skin, with the general condition and health of the skin is reflected in that colour. The efficiency of the respiration, transpiration, elimination of cellular wastes and cutaneous blood flow are all indicated by the colour of the skin. In addition, hormones, some diseases, exposure to chemicals, drugs, and temperature extremes can all cause a colour change of the skin.

 Skin conditions related to colour

- Pigmentation
- Vascular disorders
- Oxidative stress

Cells and systems involved or influenced

- Melanocyte
- Lipid peroxidation
- Keratinocyte/epidermis
- Immune system

Effective chemicals/actives

- MSH inhibitors
- L Dopa inhibitors
- Melanosome transfer inhibitors
- Anti-inflammatory
- Tyrosinase inhibitors
- Antioxidants

Skin condition: Pigmentation

There are a number of strategies pursued by all cosmetic houses to deal with pigmentation problems by the control of melanogenesis; and this market has been one of the biggest growing sections of the beauty industry.

Melanogenesis is a complex oxidative process that has a number of steps where chemical intervention can take place. However, there are a number of preparatory steps that must be taken first for effective results to be achieved. The following strategies have been separated in to preparatory and intervention categories.

The melanogenesis process

A full explanation of this fascinating process can be found in the book:
Advanced Skin Analysis
ISBN 978-0-476-00665-2

Pages 64-77

Preparatory steps:

- Improve skin barrier defence systems. (See secretions chapter)
- Improve keratinocyte cell health
- Improve the density of the spinosum layer for better distribution of melanin pigment
- Improve melanocyte dendrite length and cell membrane health with EFA's.
- Prevent lipid peroxidation with oil soluble anti-oxidants
- Ensuring lipid antioxidants are reactivated with vitamin C
- Prevent vitamin C oxidisation and replace on a daily basis.
- Prevent DNA damage with vitamin A and other similar actives.
- Include a broad-spectrum sun block to prevent further UVA & UVB stimulation of melanogenesis.
- Employ large quantities of antioxidants to prevent cell damage.

The preparatory steps are taken to clear the epidermis of incidental melanin and poor quality keratinocytes. This will ensure the epidermis is viable and has the correct density to support even distribution of melanin throughout the spinosum layer. Correct preparation will ensure better intervention results, and this may be as high as 40% with some types of epidermal pigmentation.

The next steps: intervention in the melanogenesis process

When we have a viable epidermis, the next phase of the treatment can begin.
There are five intervention points in the process that we are able to initiate change, ideally we need to address all of them simultaneously for greater effectiveness. Simply approaching one intervention point will only produce limited results. Historically, tyrosinase inhibitors were the only intervention available, but new technologies have now expanded our treatment options.

The steps in the melanogenesis process

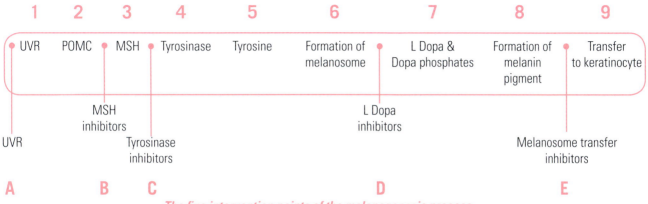

The five intervention points of the melanogenesis process

The melanogenesis process: a brief overview of cells & systems involved

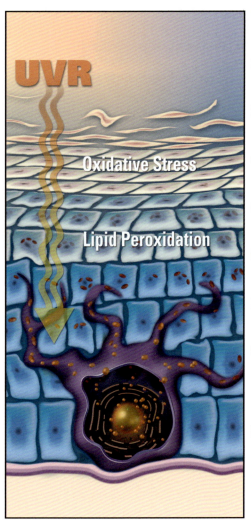

1. UVR: Primarily responsible for triggering all the subsequent steps in melanogenesis.

2. POMC: Proopiomelanocortin, formed by the pituitary gland and the precursor to the melanin-stimulating hormone (MSH).

3. Melanin stimulating hormone (MSH) adheres to the B-MICR receptor protein of the melanocytes and receptors of keratinocytes.

4. Tyrosinase: The enzyme responsible for the formation of the melanosome.

5. Tyrosine: The amino acid responsible for the formation of the melanosome.

6. Melanosome is formed by the melanocyte (Melanosome is melanin pigment carrier).

7. L Dopa & Dopa phosphates: Regulator & building blocks for the pigment melanin.

8. Melanin: The pigment responsible for the colour of the skin. There are two types: pheomelanin (red) and eumelanin (brown). Melanin is almost colourless while in the melanosome, and pigment darkening occurs after transfer to keratinocyte.

9. Melanosome is picked up by the keratinocyte via the endocytosis method, and is transported up through epidermal layers to the stratum corneum. Along the journey, it plays a role in skin barrier defence.

High risk factors for pigmentation treatments and skin lightening chemicals

Phototype 3 to 6 will have the predisposition to be at "high risk".
Always check the genetics, tanning ability and sun burn history of a client.

High risk of hyper/hypo-pigmentation after Laser/IPL treatment. Check melanin density on the treatment site before every treatment. This reading should always be referenced back to the original melanin average reading taken at the consultation or patch test appointment.
High risk for trauma, heat & chemically caused pigmentation, and moderate risk for all other pigmented skin conditions.
High risk for scarring & moderate risk for visible vascular damage.

Treatment solutions for pigmentation

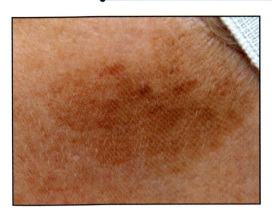

Because melanogenesis is a complicated and oxidative process in the early years it was thought that antioxidants may inhibit melanogenesis.

It was this early pathway of thinking that led to the biggest breakthroughs, this combined with a greater knowledge of melanogenesis led to better and more effective actives being developed.

Each different type of pigmented lesion has a different level of cellular damage, and in our example at left, we have a solar lentigine. The level of damage in this instance will be mitochondrial DNA damage of the melanocyte.

This level of cellular damage will mean that the melanocyte can no longer function as genetically programmed, and this will extend the treatment program time. Do not expect quick results in this instance.

As previously discussed, melanogenesis inhibitors need to address every step in the melanogenesis process for best results. We will explore each group individually.

Melanin stimulating hormone (MSH) inhibitors

By preventing the activation of the melanin stimulating hormone (MSH) receptors that are embedded in the cell membranes of both the melanocyte and keratinocytes, a reduction in all future steps of melanogenesis will occur.

Sepiwhite™ MSH inhibitor

- Also known by its INCI name of Undecylenoyl phenylalanine.
- By preventing MSH adhering to the B-MICR receptor within the cell membrane of the melanocyte and MSH receptor of the keratinocyte, all further steps in the melanogenesis process will be slowed down.

Melanostat as a MSH inhibitor

- Melanostat is a biomimetic peptide obtained by amino acid synthesis.
- By preventing MSH adhering to the B-MICR receptor within the cell membrane of the melanocyte and MSH receptor of the keratinocyte, all further steps in the melanogenesis process will be slowed down.

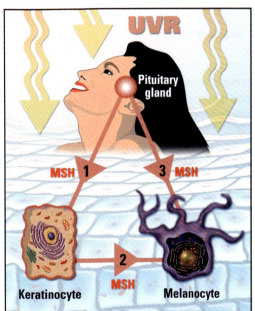

Step 1: MSH is sent from pituitary gland to keratinocyte receptor.
Step 2: Keratinocyte activates melanocyte receptor (B-MICR)
Step 3: Now that the melanocyte is activated, it can receive the MSH from the pituitary gland.

Melanostatine-5 (Aqua dextran –Nonapeptide-1) as a MSH inhibitor

• A biomimetic peptide ingredient that prevents melanocyte stimulating hormone (MSH), from adhering to the B-MICR receptor within the cell membrane of the melanocyte, slowing down all further steps in the melanogenesis process.

SulforaWhite as a MSH inhibitor

- Dual functional MSH inhibitor and antioxidant combined.
- A liposomal preparation of sulforaphane (a phytonutrient).
- By preventing MSH adhering to the B-MICR receptor within the cell membrane of the melanocyte and MSH receptor of the keratinocyte, all further steps in the melanogenesis process will be slowed down.

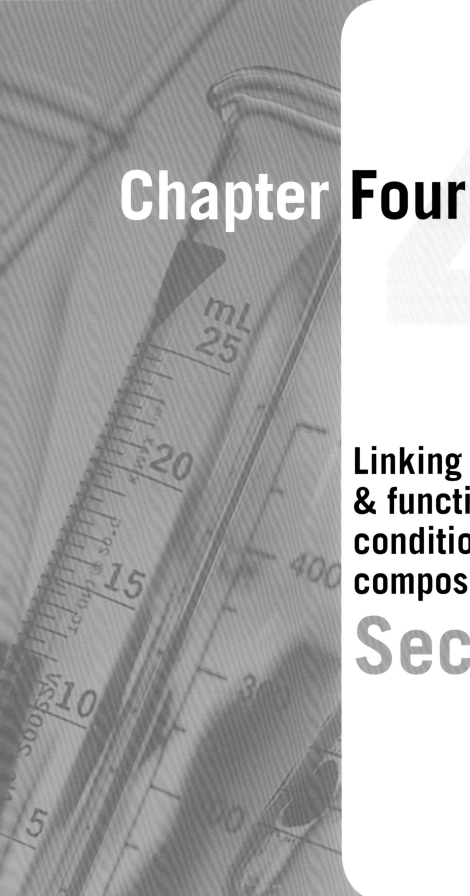

Chapter Four

Linking skin structure & function to skin condition & product composition

Secretions

Skin conditions related to secretions

Numerous factors control the secretions of the skin, some of these crossing-over from dermal to epidermal. In the same manner as with texture and colour, we will examine the two categories that influence secretions, with the external, that influences the epidermis, and the internal, that influence the dermis.

Epidermal

The fluids found on the surface of the skin, (acid mantle) are secreted from the sebaceous and sudiferous glands, in conjunction with the epidermic lipids (bilayers) and the natural moisturising factor (NMF) make up the first line of skin barrier defence.
By slowing down trans epidermal water loss the acid mantle plays a major role in retaining water, slowing evaporation thus maintaining epidermal hydration.

Dermal

The fluids of the lower levels (interstitial/extracellular) are equally important to the health of the epidermis as they are to providing support for the fibrous tissues collagen and elastin.
The hydration of these lower levels is regulated by the lymphatic and circulatory systems.
These systems work in synergy with one another to preserve fluid and nutritional balance and are a major part of the skin defence function.

Skin conditions related to secretions

- Essential fatty acid deficiency (EFAD)
- Oxidative stress
- Lipid peroxidation
- Impaired enzyme activity

Cells and systems involved or influenced

- Acid mantle
- Cell membrane
- Glycosaminoglycans
- Lipid bilayers
- Sebaceous secretion
- Amino acids

Effective chemicals/actives

- Linoleic acid
- Vitamin A
- Squalene
- Ceramides
- Alpha lipoic acid
- Alpha linolenic acid
- Phospholipids
- Sphingolipids
- Vitamin E

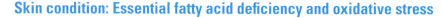

Skin condition: Essential fatty acid deficiency and oxidative stress

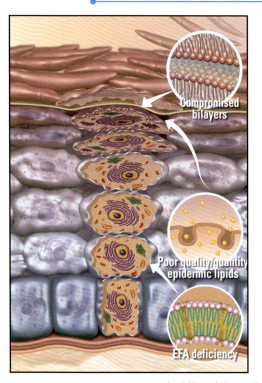

For this discussion, we are talking primarily about the keratinocyte, which is the predominant cell of the epidermis, and is primarily responsible for generating and maintaining the skin barrier defence systems of the epidermis.

During the keratinocyte's differentiation cycle, the lipid components of the cell membrane and cell interior are broken down and placed within odland bodies (small circular parcels), stored and matured for release when the cell reaches the transitional stage of the stratum lucidum.

Once released into extra cellular space, they will form bilayers that are primarily ceramides (third line of skin barrier defence) and the corneocyte (second line of skin barrier defence) will become embedded within them.

A cell will only make what it is programmed to make providing it has the nutrients to do so, therefore for a keratinocyte to form these bilayers the cell membrane needs to be in optimum condition.

Keratinocytes have around 45% phospholipids as part of the cell membrane, and it has been firmly established that the phospholipids require 4% essential fatty acids to remain lipophilic and to form the ceramide 1 component of the bilayers.

Lipid peroxidation is one of the most severe types of damage that can occur to a cell membrane: this is when all lipid antioxidants are lost and not restored in a cell membrane and the phospholipid component is compromised.

Once the cell membrane has been compromised, intracellular oxidative stress may easily occur, leading to mitochondria DNA damage of a cell and the resulting inability of that cell to function efficiently.

It is a combination of oxidative stress and EFAD that accelerates the loss of oil-soluble antioxidants such as vitamin E, and in conjunction with the oxidisation of vitamin C, leads to lipid peroxidation.

Maintaining the active and passive ability of cell membranes will lead to the prevention of many basic skin conditions and disorders.

The following mono and polyunsaturated lipids are those that are found throughout the "skin lipids" of the epidermis; however these are not all of the lipids of the epidermis. Triglycerides, neutral lipids and free fatty acids etc have not been included in this exercise as they are not classified as biomimetic actives.

EFA metabolism

The 4% essential fatty acid component that is required to maintain the phospholipid component of a cell membrane is not metabolised and the only source is via the diet or being topically applied.
(See pages 26-27)

Many books have been written about the nutritional benefits of essential fatty acids, and some innovative skin care companies are now including these essential fats into cosmetic formulations.

Cell membrane composition	Bilayers composition	Skin surface lipids	Free lipids of the epidermis
Phospholipids	Ceramides	Squalene	ßeta-carotene
Squalene	Sphingolipids	Ceramides	Squalene
Sphingolipids	Squalene	Glucosylceramides	Alpha lipoic acid
Glucosylceramides	Phospholipids		Retinyl palmitate
Ceramides			
Linoleic acid			
Alpha linolenic acid			
Vitamin E			
Alpha lipoic acid			

Treatment solutions: EFAD and oxidative stress

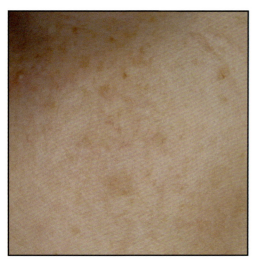

Lipofuscins are a visual result of EFAD and lipid peroxidation including glycation of cell membrane proteins.

When addressing skin conditions of the epidermis where lipid dryness and compromised acid mantle are present, these are outward indicators that lipid based skin barrier defence systems are no longer functioning correctly.
To effectively supplement these missing lipids with biomimetic substances we must understand the lipid components of a cell membrane, the acid mantle and epidermic lipids. This is the first step towards linking skin structure and function to product composition, and we need to look for what ingredients are available that will match each of the epidermic lipids and these will be found among the world of plants, algae's, seeds, and if required, synthetics.

Phospholipids

The most often used material for the production of phospholipids has been lecithin; a phospholipid/oil mixture that today is almost exclusively extracted from soybeans. We discussed in the first chapter of this book the role that soybean lecithin plays in the formation of liposomes as a cosmetic formulation delivery system for other actives. The compatibility that liposomes have for skin lipids and cell membranes of the epidermis is well known by clinicians that have undertaken cosmetic chemistry training with me in the past.

Phosphatidylcholine (INCI lecithin) and phospholipids

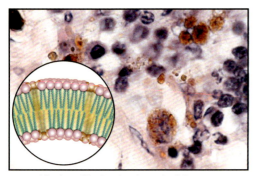

Histology slide showing glycated cellular waste known as lipofuscin

Another component of lecithin is phosphatidylcholine, sometimes abbreviated as PC. Unlike its base substance lecithin, when phosphatidylcholine is mixed with water it spontaneously generates cell-like structures.
This structure is built up in bilayers just like in natural cell structure of the epidermal skin barrier defence systems. (These would have similar structure to the liposomes previously discussed in chapter one).

What is more exciting is that the phosphatidylcholine of the membranes contains two substances in chemically combined form which are essential for the skin, and which cannot be metabolised; linoleic acid and choline. (See side bar)
While the choline component takes over skin protection functions and plays an important role in the prevention of skin ageing, the linoleic acid component improves the natural barrier function of the skin on a long-term basis by integrating into ceramide I. There is also a direct correlation between prostaglandin 3 (PG3) and omega 3 (alpha-linolenic acid) in the reduction of cellular inflammation.

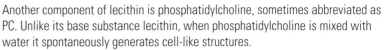

Choline

Choline is an organic compound, classified as a water-soluble essential nutrient and usually grouped within the Vitamin B complex. This natural amine is found in the lipids that make up cell membranes.

Squalene

Cosmetic sources of squalene exhibit the same properties as epidermic squalene, and so penetrate the skin quickly. Squalene is not very susceptible to peroxidation and appears to function in the skin as a quencher of singlet oxygen radical, protecting the skin from lipid peroxidation caused by sunburn and oxidative stress.
Botanic sources of squalene are rice bran, wheat germ, olives, amaranth seed and also from shark liver oil. In the cosmetic industry it is becoming increasingly less acceptable to use animal sourced ingredients, and there has been a continual move towards all plant-based derivatives, biomimetic synthetics and ingredients that have more compatibility with skin layers and lipids.

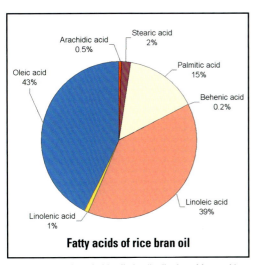

Fatty acids of rice bran oil

When looking for suitable oil, the distribution of fatty acids is important. The high percentage of linoleic acid (omega 6) in rice bran oil is highly beneficial to skin health, although the high oleic acid content (43%) would make it unsuitable for active, oily, acneic skins.

Rice bran oil (Oryza sativa) as a source of squalene

Next to palm oil, rice bran oil is probably one of the most useful commodities in the cosmetic world, not just because of its compatibility, but also because it is considered a renewable resource.

As a vitamin E source, rice bran oil is rich not only in alpha tocopherol but also has the highest amount of tocotrienols in liquid form vegetable oils.

It also contains the less known antioxidant oryzanol. Cosmetic formulators recognise rice bran oil's oxidative stability and have been investigating the reports that oryzanol has an ability to reduce erythema caused by sunburn. There are many plant sources of oil that have compatibility with the skin, with many suitable for body products, however few have the matching criteria for skin lipids.

Derivatives of rice bran come in many forms from oils that we know as extracts, waxes, powders, fatty acids, hydrolysed proteins and the use throughout the cosmetic industry is very wide. Commonly found as a surfactant, emulsifier, abrasives, binders and emollients in skin care and personal care products.

Amaranth caudatus seed oil as a source of squalene

Amaranth caudatus is almost the only plant showing a high concentration of squalene (2.4 to 8.0%) compared to other vegetable oils. In addition, to having a high percentage of tocopherols and tocotrienols, amaranths caudatus contains linoleic acid. This oil exhibits very good anti-inflammatory effects, is non-comedogenic and suitable for treating dry, itchy skin as well as eczema and psoriasis.

Olive oil as a source of squalene

Olive oil contains the largest percentage of squalene among the common vegetable oils. For instance, olive oil has 136-708 mg/100g of squalene. Olive oil is composed mainly of the mixed triglyceride esters of oleic acid and palmitic acid and of other fatty acids and sterols (about 0.2% phytosterol and tocosterols).

Sphingolipids

Yeast as a source of sphingolipids

Amide

In chemistry, amide usually refers to organic compounds that contain the specific groups of atoms consisting of an Acyl group (C=O) linked to a nitrogen atom (N)

Ceramide is the fundamental structural unit common to all sphingolipids. They consist simply of a fatty acid chain attached through an amide linkage to sphingosine. It is very difficult to isolate highly pure ceramides, regardless of origin, animal or plant. Sphingolipids sourced from the yeast ***pichia ciferrii*** have shown to have compatibility with skin and have been successfully exploited to produce certain types of ceramides in large quantities.

- Sphingomyelins have a phosphorylcholine or phosphoroethanolamine molecule with an ether linkage to the 1-hydroxy group of a ceramide.
- Glycosphingolipids differ in the substituents on their head group, and are ceramides with one or more sugar residues joined in a -glycosidic linkage at the 1-hydroxyl position.

Ceramides and glucosylceramides

Ceramides are a major component of the bilayers of the stratum corneum by weight (Ceramides 1 to 7). We have read many times that the ceramide 1 is ester linked to linoleic acid and about the benefits of the stratum corneum lipids like cholesterol sulphate and fatty acids in maintaining skin barrier defence systems.

Glucosylceramides are a precursor to the ceramide group and are part of the differentiation of the keratinocyte's life cycle, and the formation of odland bodies that store and mature the epidermic lipids of the bilayers. See chapter one for details of various forms of ceramides.

Pro-Lipiskin INCI name: pichia anomala extract (yeast)

- This ingredient has shown to boost the epidermic lipids of the bilayers by acting on the key steps such as synthesis, transport, secretion and maturation of epidermic lipids.
- The bilayers are improved, therefore ensuring better skin barrier defence, and as a result, trans-epidermal water loss is reduced.
- A good example of biomimetic moisturisers of the new millennium.

Omega-3 Ceramide

- A linseed oil/ palm oil aminopropanediol ester.
- An alpha-linoleic acid stabilised under a ceramide-like structure.
- Obtained from flax oil by a patented enzymatic solvent free process.

Omega-6 ceramides

- A group of omega-6 ceramide-like molecules obtained by the same enzymatic process as omega 3 ceramides.
- Hybrid palm oil aminopropanediol esters with wheat germ, cottonseed, and evening primrose oil.

Alpha linolenic & linoleic & (Omega 3 & 6)

Essential fatty acids are necessary for maintaining the viability of the phospholipids of the keratinocyte cell membrane and for the formation of prostaglandin's PGE1, PGE2 and PGE3, ceramides, acid mantle, and bilayers. We will begin with alpha linolenic acid. (Omega 3 or n-3)

The major sources of omega 3 that would be used in the cosmetic industry for facial creams are hemp seed oil, flax seed oil and soybean oil.

Fish oil is widely used as a supplement and some fish roe and algae are used as sources of omega 3, with spirulina an example.

Kiwi oil as a source of alpha linolenic acid (INCI: Actinidia chinensis)

- High content of alpha linolenic acid, (ALA), the main omega 3 essential fatty acid found in plant and fruit seed lipids.
- Typically contains around 61% ALA, which is higher than many of the other conventional oils commercially available. (e.g. flax, camelina, hemp, walnut oil)

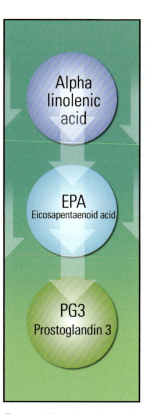

The matabolic pathway of omega 3 See page 27 for full details.

More information can be found in pages 122-126 of the Advanced Skin Analysis book

Camelina oil as a source of alpha linolenic acid

- Also known as 'Gold of pleasure' or false flax.
- Approx 40% of oil is rich in omega 3 fatty acids.
- Under independent skin studies, camelina oil was found to be an ideal treatment medium for EFAD and impaired acid mantles.

Hemp seed oil as a source of linoleic and alpha linolenic acid

- Extracted from special variety of hemp.
- Good natural source of the essential fatty acids, alpha linolenic acid (Omega 3) and linoleic acid (Omega 6).
- Good skin protection properties and particularly useful in the treatment of lipid dry skin and essential fatty acid deficiency.

Borage seed oil as a source of linoleic acid

- Derived from the seeds of the Borago officinalis plant, it has one of the highest amounts of gamma-linolenic acid (Omega-6) of seed oils.
- Exhibits anti-inflammatory properties, and is suitable for impaired acid mantles, EFAD and some forms of dermatitis.

Evening primrose oil (EPO) as a source of linoleic acid

- Contains EFA gamma-linolenic acid (Omega 6) and low amount of linoleic acid. (Omega 3)
- Emollient properties make it suitable for use in formulas that hydrate and soften the skin.
- Vitamin E is often added to the oil to prevent oxidation during storage and processing.

Biomimetic epidermic lipids

Alpha lipoic acid (ALA) (INCI: Thioctic acid) as an epidermic lipid

- This very small molecule can pass freely through the cell membrane and works in synergy with vitamins C, E and ßeta-carotene.
- Thioctic acid is a unique antioxidant and protector of all cells because it is the only nutrient which is both oil and water soluble.
- A coenzyme in the metabolic process for the conversion of glucose to energy, (ATP) making it an important part of a cell's mitochondria.
- Thioctic acids found in cosmetics are of synthetic origin.

ßeta-carotene and retinyl palmitate as an epidermic lipid

- ßeta-carotene is primarily used as an antioxidant and will work in synergy with other vitamins such as vitamins C and E.
- Both ßeta-carotene and retinyl palmitate are found in large quantities throughout the epidermis.
- Both of these vitamin A esters will be easily assimilated into the epidermic lipids when topically applied.
- Studies have shown that up to 44% of the absorbed retinyl palmitate was hydrolysed to retinol, indicating that the use of retinyl palmitate in cosmetic formulations may result in significant delivery of retinol into the skin.

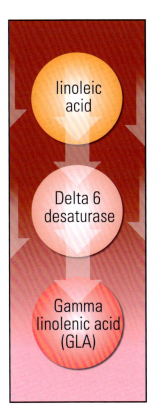

linoleic acid

Delta 6 desaturase

Gamma linolenic acid (GLA)

The matabolic pathway of omega 6
See page 27 for full details.

More information can be found in pages 122-126 of the Advanced Skin Analysis book

Skin condition: Lipid peroxidation

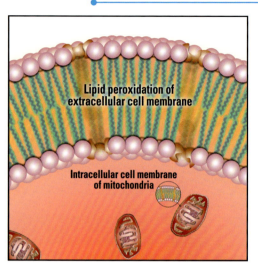

Lipid peroxidation of extracellular cell membrane

Intracellular cell membrane of mitochondria

This is a skin condition that is linked to oxidative stress, and like most skin conditions that are associated with secretions of the skin, can be classified as a "secondary cause." By this, I mean one step after the leading cause, which in this case is oxidative stress or in simpler client language "free radicals".

Lipid peroxidation refers to the oxidative degradation of lipids, and is the process whereby free radicals `steal' electrons from the molecules of phospholipids in cell membranes, resulting in cell damage. When the cell membranes become compromised, loss of membrane integrity results.

The loss of oil-soluble antioxidants happens almost simultaneously as the loss of water-soluble antioxidants. This is because they work in synergy, and so you must consider replacing both. You can't think of one without thinking of the other. In simple terms vitamin E (oil soluble) needs vitamin C (water soluble) to become reactivated.

Treatment solutions: Lipid peroxidation

Lipid peroxidation is not just the loss of oil soluble antioxidants; it is the attack on the phospholipid content of the cell membrane that results in reduced permeability and active and passive transfer of nutrients and waste, including the glycation of cell membrane lipids. This will compound into lipofuscin and/or intracellular oxidative stress.
Lipid peroxidation also occurs at the mitochondrial membranes, degrading cardiolipin, (See sidebar) changing the mitochondrial membrane potential, eventually leading to possible cell self-destruction/death. (Apoptosis)
All of the same oil-soluble antioxidants that were recommended for pigmentation lipid peroxidation are again utilised here, with some additions under the carotene family.

DMAE (Dimethylaminoethanol)

- DMAE is an analog of the B vitamin, choline, (a water-soluble essential nutrient) and a precursor of acetylcholine. (A cytokine-like molecule that regulates basic cellular processes such as proliferation, differentiation, movement and secretion) It also exhibits moderately active anti-inflammatory properties.
- A powerful antioxidant that has the ability to combine with radicals to bind them before they can do damage to skin cells. (A little like a spin-trap)
- Molecular structure allows it to insert itself between components of the cell plasma membrane to help protect and keep the cell membrane intact
- Inhibits production of arachidonic acid and other chemicals responsible for pain and cellular inflammation.

Super dismutase oxide (SOD)

- Manganese super dismutase oxide (Mn SOD) protects the mitochondria from free radical damage.
- The body needs plenty of vitamin C and copper to make this natural antioxidant.
- Super dismutase is part of the intracellular antioxidant brigade, therefore making it a "must have" antioxidant for any skin condition, not just lipid peroxidation.

Cardiolipin

(IUPAC name "1,3-bis(sn-3'-phosphatidyl)-sn-glycerol") is an important component of the inner mitochondrial membrane, where it constitutes about 20% of the total lipid composition. Cardiolipin (CL) is found almost exclusively in the inner mitochondrial membrane where it is essential for the optimal function of numerous enzymes that are involved in mitochondrial energy metabolism.

Ergothioneine (EGT), also called thioneine

- L- ergothioneine is a stable antioxidant found in plants and animal tissue.
- It has proven to be efficient in inhibiting lipid peroxidation formation by scavenging radicals and protecting cells from UV induced ROS.
- Keratinocytes have receptors for ergothioneine and can internalise it. The receptor is the door to get into the cell: therefore, it is believed that ergothioneine can be utilized within the cell.
- Different than many antioxidants that only work around the extracellular area, ergothioneine can penetrate the cell.
- This antioxidant formulates well with sun protection chemicals and will prove to be very beneficial in all forms of skin care.
- Potential to become as popular as ascorbic acid. Its major point of difference, apart from being a biomimetic active as an antioxidant, is that it donates electrons to molecules that need them.

Vitamin E

Working in synergy with vitamin C, the vitamin E family is necessary for the prevention of lipid peroxidation, thus preserving the integrity of the cell membrane of the dendritic melanocyte.

Tocotrienols

Some research suggests tocotrienols are more potent in their anti-oxidation effect than the common forms of tocopherol due to significant differences in chemical structure.

ßeta-carotene

Being an oil soluble vitamin give ßeta-carotene the ability to meld with all of the oil phases of the acid mantle, bilayers and cell membranes, making this simple active invaluable in the treatment and prevention of lipid peroxidation.

Alpha lipoic acid (ALA) (Thioctic acid)

Alpha lipoic acid works together with other antioxidants such as vitamins C and E. What this means is that when vitamin E quenches lipid peroxidation a vitamin E radical is formed and that radical is reduced back to vitamin E by lipoic acid. It does a similar task with vitamin C, in turn vitamin C can also reduce vitamin E.

Lycopene

A very powerful quencher of the singlet oxygen radical, which is one of the reactive oxygen species (ROS) linked to oxidation of cell membrane lipids. Lycopene is found in many fruits and vegetables especially high in tomatoes and goji berries. Not only are goji berries rich in several vitamins and minerals, they have been rated number one on the Oxygen Radical Absorbance Capacity (ORAC) scale, which measures the antioxidant levels in food.

I expect we will see many skin care lines with antioxidants that have origins of the goji berry and similar lycopene based plants in the future.

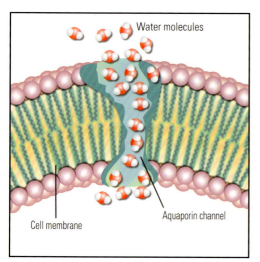

Aquaporins control much of the water that passes through in to a cell. There are similar receptors on the cell membrane for nutrients and hormones. Substances that are compatible to the aquaporin channel will be the saturating and hydrating actives of the future.

Water solubles of the epidermis (Natural moisturising factor or NMF)

The water content of the epidermal layers varies considerably, with the basal layer around 70% and significantly less in the outermost layer. (Approx 13% for a correctly functioning stratum corneum)

To some extent, other factors such as the relevant ambient humidity, the lipid phases of the bilayers, and an intact acid mantle regulate this amount. The water phase of the basal layer is more concentrated with substances like hyaluronic acid that has seeped through the dermal/epidermal junction, and this fluid surrounds the active cells within that layer.

Hyaluronic acid is not found higher up in the epidermis because it is believed that its heavy molecular weight causes it to stay within the bottom of the epidermis and therefore not evaporate with the rest of the water solubles.

Forty percent of the water phase of the epidermis is amino acids, and these as a group, are believed to be important contributors to stratum corneum hydration.

Importance of the water phase of the epidermis

Water regulates all bodily functions, including the activities of circulating and dissolving. Every hydrophilic enzymatic and chemical reaction of the body occurs in the presence of water.

We know that the primary source of water to the skin is via fluid intake; therefore the client is responsible for the hydration of the skin. This is why I referred to this as a "secondary cause" in the Advanced Skin Analysis book, and by this I meant the therapist should be targeting more important issues within the skin than chasing water (eg. rebuilding the oil phases to slow water evaporation). So much emphasis is placed on hydration and dehydration of the epidermis, that it has become a primary target for those that market cosmetics, to those that sell them, and of course the end user. There has been so much emphasis that I believe we have lost our way as a profession, and that we need to think more like formulatory chemists to find our way back. I use this next paragraph as an example of what I mean.

Mask before Massage

Of all of the procedures that are used in treating impaired enzyme activity, (dehydration in the old terms) the facial where the combination of a mask and massage is used needs to be revised from the "old methods" employed by many aestheticians and therapists. This is the sequence of facial mask and massage.

The skin care products used during a facial treatment, (irrespective of the skin condition) are all, if not 99% are water-soluble. This means that every step saturates and hydrates the upper layers of the epidermis; i.e. stratum corneum and the transitional upper granulosum.

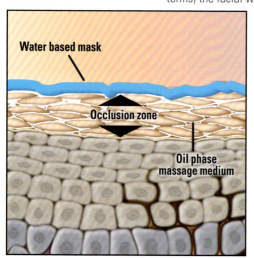

The only oil phase commonly used is the massage medium, and a majority of aestheticians and beauty therapists are taught that it should be placed on the skin before the mask.

If the massage medium is oil based, how is it possible for a water-based mask to effectively infiltrate into the epidermis post massage, now that the skin has been partially occluded?

This must be remembered when any infusion of ingredients to restore the water phase of the epidermis is undertaken. Logically, any oil based massage should be the *final* step in any treatment.

Treatment solutions for lack of free water and impaired enzyme activity

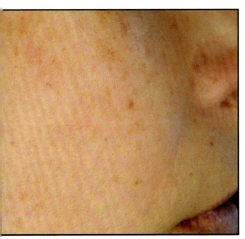

The primary cause of this skin condition is EFAD, which has compromised the acid mantle, and in turn has accelerated the onset of diffused redness. This combined with fast TEWL has caused crystalisation of epidermic lipids and poor quality bilayers with low ceramide content.

This skin condition has one thing in common with essential fatty acid deficiency, and this is the basic primary cause is due to deficiencies in the clients fluid/dietary intake. For any treatment regime or product to be successful, this primary cause must be addressed by increasing fluid intake and restoring sufficient quantity of skin lipids to reduce the fast evaporation of water.

This is just typical of how your mindset must be; never think of water without remembering that oil is part of the equation, and this applies to both the skin and to cosmetic formations.

We will begin this next segment by covering those water soluble humectants and film formers that have an affinity with the epidermis. We will then look at the substances that have compatibility with the dermis.

Epidermal, dermal & intracellular compatible humectants

Sodium Pyrrolidone carboxylic acid (Na PCA) as part of the NMF

- Na PCA is found in the stratum corneum natural moisturising factor at about 4%, and this sodium salt is more hygroscopic than glycerin. (Refer page 15, chapter 1 as a humectant in emulsions.)
- The hygroscopic action of attracting water from the air plus an excellent hydrophilic ability of being able to absorb several times its weight in water makes Na PCA an excellent humectant, with a saturation ability.
- Leaves more NMF behind in the skin than it takes, and can mimic the water-solubles already present in the epidermis.

Amino Acids

- Amino acids totalling 40% of the stratum corneum are some of the most popular cosmetic ingredients; their normal presence in skin contributes to their attractiveness.
- Some of these acids are derived directly from the hydrolysis of protein, and the biggest amino acid pool supply seems to be filaggrin, which is hydrolysed as the differentiating keratinocytes complete the keratinisation process.
- Amino acids have become the basis of the popular peptide ingredients, and it is well accepted that as a group they are considered to be important contributors to stratum corneum hydration. Many algae and plants are used as a basis and contribute to the amino acids used and synthesized by formulators today.

Sericin (silk amino acids)

- Sericin is often marketed as silk amino acids, so when reading cosmetic labels or literature you may only see one or the other of these words.
- Sericin, AKA silk amino acids, give the skin a very soft and velvety feel when used in a cosmetic product, and have some excellent water-binding properties, with some antioxidant action.
- The range of amino acids that are part of this compound is extensive, including 18 kinds of amino acids, with L-alanine, L-serine and glycine accounting for over 80% of the total.

- Silk amino acids are quickly absorbed, taking part in the enzyme activity of the epidermis, improving other epidermal functions, including antioxidant properties and effective treating of lipid peroxidation.
- Sericin is a tyrosinase inhibitor, and is one of the few actives able to reduce the MMP collagenase enzymes that are increased by sun exposure. (Effectively treats three skin conditions)

Glutathione

- An important intracellular antioxidant that protects against a variety of different radical species and is a compound classified as a tripeptide made of three amino acids, cysteine, glutamic acid and glycine.
- Works in synergy with vitamin C within the water phase of the cell as well as the cell membrane.

Calcium & magnesium

- This essential element regulates cell turnover of the keratinocyte, regulates lipid formation of the bilayers and plays a role in reducing cellular inflammation.
- An integral part of the water solubles (NMF) 1.5% within the stratum corneum and in higher quantities in the lower layers where the cell membrane is permeable with aquaporins where ion receptors function for calcium, magnesium and potassium etc.
- Calcium comes to the beauty industry in several ways, high levels of these elements are found in bentonite clay-based masks that are rich in 70 trace minerals and essential for skin health.

Chitin

- Chitin and its derivatives allow active principles to be placed in close contact with the skin by means of a medium that is not only a film-forming tensor, but is especially saturating.
- This is a new double advantage that makes chitin of great value as an integral ingredient used in skin care products.
- Chitin facilitates the effects of other hydrating agents: solar filters, organic acids or other active principles can be combined with the derivatives of chitin.

Chitin nanofibrils

- Chitin has now been developed into nanofibrils and therefore is able to link active compounds via hydrogen bonds and as a result increase penetration into skin layers.
- These nanofibrils have been deployed into improving photo protection and anti-inflammatory compounds in sun protection products.

ßeta-glucans

- Oat ßeta-glucan has a long history of safe use in skin care and dermatology as a long-lasting, film-forming humectant. It has also been shown to work as an anti-irritant and to speed up healing of shallow abrasions and partial thickness burns.
- Products containing purified oat ßeta-glucan (rather than whole oatmeal) do exist but are few.
- Also, they are hard to compare as they rarely have ßeta-glucan concentration stated on the label.
- It is unclear whether products with colloidal oatmeal would contain sufficient amounts of oat ßeta-glucan, but it is known that oatmeal has saturating and anti-inflammatory benefits on lipid dry skins.
- ßeta-glucans also formulate well with sun protection products.

Glucosamine as a supporting dermal reserve fluid

Glucosamine

When combined with niacinamide (B3), N-acetyl glucosamine has proven to be an excellent treatment of pigmentation.

- This element is found within the basal layer of the epidermis and is the building block for larger molecules such as hyaluronic acid, which forms part of the dermal reserve.
- Because glucosamine is the precursor of hyaluronic acid, increasing levels of the former could lead to a corresponding increase in production of hyaluronic acid.
- In addition, because keratinocytes continually make and break down HA, the ability to be able to increase epidermal levels from topical application of glucosamine would be an added bonus to the health of the epidermis.
- High quality glucosamine is produced by microbial fermentation; however marine based (shells of lobster, shrimp and crab) sources are also used.
- Glucosamine HCL, (glucosamine hydrochloride) acetyl glucosamine (a monosaccharide derivative) and ascorbyl glucosamine (glucosamine combined with L- ascorbic acid) are common forms available.

Hyaluronic acid (HA), sodium hyaluronate as a supporting dermal reserve fluid

- Hyaluronic acid and its salts are members of the non-protein class of glycosaminoglycans. (GAGS)
- HA is also offered as a high molecular weight, hydrophillic material that functions as a "molecular sponge", allowing for extensive hydration.
- Film forming and hydrophilic properties, in addition to high molecular weight make for good humectant characteristics. (Saturation)
- HA can also function as a transdermal delivery system for other "actives" since it forms a matrix on the skin, allowing increased skin penetration due to skin saturation and hydration.
- Modern variants from sterile, bio-fermentation extraction processes, (synthetic) and "natural" animal sources (rooster-comb and bovine ocular-material) are available.

Urea as part of the natural moisturising factor (NMF)

- Urea is present at about 1.0 to 1.5% in the stratum corneum, and is formed by the amino acid arginine and from the eccrine sweat gland. Quantities vary in each individual; it is very hygroscopic and still used in creams in percentages as high as 20%.
- Urea is keratolytic and its benefits for long-term use as skin care have been questioned due to cellular dehiscence (swelling & bursting) of corneocytes.
- Any prolonged use combined with lipid dryness (very common) causes a reduction in the density of the spinosum layer; this combined with increased desquamation caused by the keratolytic ability of urea increases water evaporation (TEWL) through the epidermis.
- One of the more beneficial uses of urea is that it exhibits broad-spectrum antibacterial properties, and when a urea-based cream is applied for a short time to open, compromised and broken elderly skin it reduces the side effect of possible secondary infection while the epidermic heals.
- Unfortunately the short-term benefits that people often experience soon disappear, and often the original skin dryness returns, but worse.

Florence says:

This page is the final lesson in understanding how product composition can link to skin structure and function, followed by how those two things are linked to a skin condition.

When writing up a treatment program for clinical and home care use, place the primary cause as part of the correction pathway into the clients homework.

Then place the damaged cells and systems into the clinical treatment pathway.

Choosing products with ingredients that have a synergy to those damaged cells and systems is the first step in raising the chances that the treatment regime and home care products will be successful.

Impaired enzyme activity & intra/extracellular fluids : Chemical treatment solutions

Product characteristics & suitability	Compromised skin	High risk skin	Impaired acid mantle	Anti-inflammatory	Lipid peroxidation	Oxidative stress	Antioxidant	NMF epidermis	Intracellular	Dermal reserve	Hygroscopic	Humectant	Saturating/ film forming	Water soluble	Peptides
NaPCA	✓	✓	✓	✓		✓		✓	✓			✓	✓	✓	
Amino acids	✓	✓	✓	✓	✓	✓		✓	✓	✓		✓	✓	✓	
Sericin (silk amino acids)	✓	✓	✓	✓	✓			✓	✓			✓	✓	✓	✓
Glutathione	✓	✓	✓	✓	✓	✓	✓	✓	✓	✓		✓	✓	✓	
Calcium	✓	✓	✓	✓	✓	✓		✓	✓			✓	✓	✓	
Magnesium	✓	✓	✓	✓	✓	✓		✓	✓			✓	✓	✓	
Chitin	✓	✓	✓	✓				✓	✓	✓		✓	✓	✓	
Chitin nanofibrils	✓	✓	✓	✓				✓	✓	✓		✓	✓	✓	✓
ßeta-glucan	✓	✓	✓	✓				✓	✓	✓		✓	✓	✓	
Urea								✓			✓	✓		✓	
Glucosamine	✓	✓	✓	✓	✓	✓	✓	✓	✓	✓		✓	✓	✓	
Hyaluronic acid	✓	✓	✓	✓	✓	✓		✓	✓	✓		✓	✓	✓	

(Row group label, left side vertical: Epidermal & dermal compatible humectants)

In summary

You may have remembered reading where I said there is a repeat pattern and synergy in skin physiology and cosmetic chemistry; the synergy takes many forms throughout skin and chemistry especially among vitamins and how they work together.

An example is vitamin C reactivating E within the cell membrane, and as you familiarise yourself with cosmetic formulations, you will always see these two vitamins together; one as the antioxidant of the other.

The same synergy of oil and water is apparent from the cell membrane through the epidermis to the bilayers of the stratum corneum and acid mantle. For the bilayers of the epidermis to remain smooth and lipophillic, a percentage of water must be within the bilayer structure to do this.

For the sebaceous and sudiferous secretions to blend together into the acid mantle, the ceramides of the bilayers are present to play the role of the emulsifier/surfactant, and as you have learned in a skin care formulation, a surfactant is required to keeps the phases of a cream together.

Just like the acid mantle will not be properly formed without the emulsification ability of ceramides, a cosmetic cream will not remain stable without an emulsifier.
As you can see, there are parallels with how a good skin care product works and the natural chemical occurrences of the skin.

I hope this book has helped bring to you more understanding and knowledge of how important and wonderful the world of cosmetic chemistry can be.
During your basic training you probably often wondered why you had to learn so much anatomy and physiology. My book on advanced skin analysis certainly put that into perspective didn't it?

Well now, that knowledge also has to be carried into the world of cosmetic chemistry.

To stay true to the Pastiche Method; Link skin condition to skin structure and function, and logically extend this to linking skin structure and function to product composition.

Enjoy your new knowledge. Share and use it wisely.

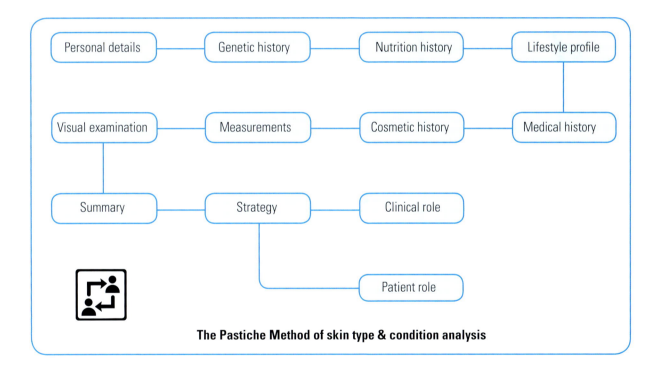

The Pastiche Method of skin type & condition analysis

References used in this book

[1] K D Marenus, PhD, "Functional Ultrastructure of the Epidermis" Cosmetic & Toiletries, vol 99, 52, 1984.

[2] Martin M Rieger, PhD, "Keratinocyte Function" Cosmetic & Toiletries, vol 107, 35-40 1992

[3] Jean L Bolognia & Seth J Orlow, "Melanocyte Biology" Pigmentary Disorders. Page 44.

[4] Derek R Highley, PhD, "The Epidermal Keratinization Process" vol 99, 60-61

[5] Martin Rieger, PhD, "Skin Constituents as Cosmetic Ingredients", vol 107 89-90 1992.

[6] Rolf D Petersen, PhD, "Ceramides Key Components for Skin Protection" vol 107, 45-49

[7] Scientifi c Backgrounders, "Alpha Lipoic Acid", page 2, HYPERLINK "http://www.nnfa.org/services/science/bg" www.nnfa.org/services/science/bg, March 19th 2003.

[8] Alpha-Lipoic Acid 1-3, HYPERLINK "http://www.usadrug.com" www.usadrug.com 19th March 2004

[9] "Some substances which cause photosensitivity", National Occupational health & Safety Commission, www.geocities.com/fragranceallergy

[10] The Healing Wound, "Inflammatory Phase", www.greenfingerslandscaping.com/wounds/html/woundhealing1.htm 26th march
2004

[11] Eugene P Pittz PhD, "Skin Barrier Function & use of Cosmetics", Cosmetic & Toiletries, Vol 99, Dec 1984.

[12] "Omega 6 & 3 Essential Fatty Acids" (Evening Primrose and Fish Oils) 1-2 HYPERLINK "http://www.enerex.bc.ca/omega_6and_3.htm" www.enerex.bc.ca/omega_6and_3.htm 26th March 2004

[13] Vitamin E delivery system, Australian biotechnology Phosphagenics, www.cosmeticdesign-europe.com Katie Bird, 03 August 2009-10-26

[14] By Murad Alam, Hayes B. Gladstone, Rebecca Tung. Cosmetic Dermatology. Publisher Elsevier Health Sciences, 2008 ISBN 0702031437,9780702031434

[15] Vitamin C and Vitamin A by Dr Des Fernandes Plastic Surgeon, Environ, South Africa

[16] A Consumer Dictionary of Cosmetic Ingredients (Third Edition) (Ruth Winter) ISBN 978-1-4000-5233-2

[17] Milady's Skin Care and Cosmetics Ingredients Dictionary (Third Edition) (Natalia Michalun, M. Varinia Michalun) ISBN 978-1-4354-8020-9

[18] Advanced Professional Skin Care, Medical Edition Peter T, Pugliese, MD ISBN 978-0-9630-2113-7

[19] Dr Lance Setterfield MD, Cosmetic vs. Medical Needling Revisited, Aesthetic "Mesotherapy", Controversies in Aesthetic Medicine, Combination Therapy. 13th July 2009.

[20] P J Stewart, "A new Image of the Periodic Table', Education in Chemistry, 41 (6) 156-158, November 2004

[21] P J Steward 'A Century on the Dmitrii Mendeleev: Tables And Spirals, 'Noble Gases and Nobel Prizes', Foundations of Chemistry, 9 (3), 00.235-245, October 2007.

[22] Hitesh Chavda, Aquaporins: The secret highways for water transport
www.pharmainfo.info.net/reviews/aquaporines-secret-files 11th April 2008

[23] Bud Brewster, C&T magazine, Aquaporins: stimulation by vitamins and sugar alcohols www.cosmetic&toiletries.com

[24] Frances J Storrs Allergen of the year: Fragrance. www.medscap.com/viewarticle/559985

[25] FDA, Colour Addditive Status List. www.fda.gov February 2009-10-26

[26] Katie Bird, Formulation and Science, Preservatives, www.cosmeticsdesign-europe.com 27th August 2009-10-26

[27] Singera, Feniol, www.sinerga.it

[28] Salinaturals, Essential oils extracts from antural plant source blended in synergistic combination can preserve cosmetic and personal care formulations www.salinaturals.com

[29] Fred Khoury, Green Chemistry. Research & Development, Above Rinaldi Labs, Inc. www.aboverinaldilabs.com

[30] Microencapsulated whitening complex, Soliance, Cosmetic & Toiletries www.cosmeticandtoiletries.com

[31] Pierfrancesco Morganti. Chitan for improved photoprotection. Cosmetics & Toiletries. Volume124. No9. September 2009

[32] Howard J Maibach MD, Peptides for aged skin. Cosmetics & Toiletries. Volume124. No9. September 2009

[33] Julie K Salmon MD. Generation Z antioxidants. Cosmetics & Toiletries. Volume124. No8. August 2009

[34] David C Steinburg. Labeling Claims. Cosmetics & Toiletries. Volume124. No8. August 2009

[35] Cosmetic chemistry references. www.cosmetics.org

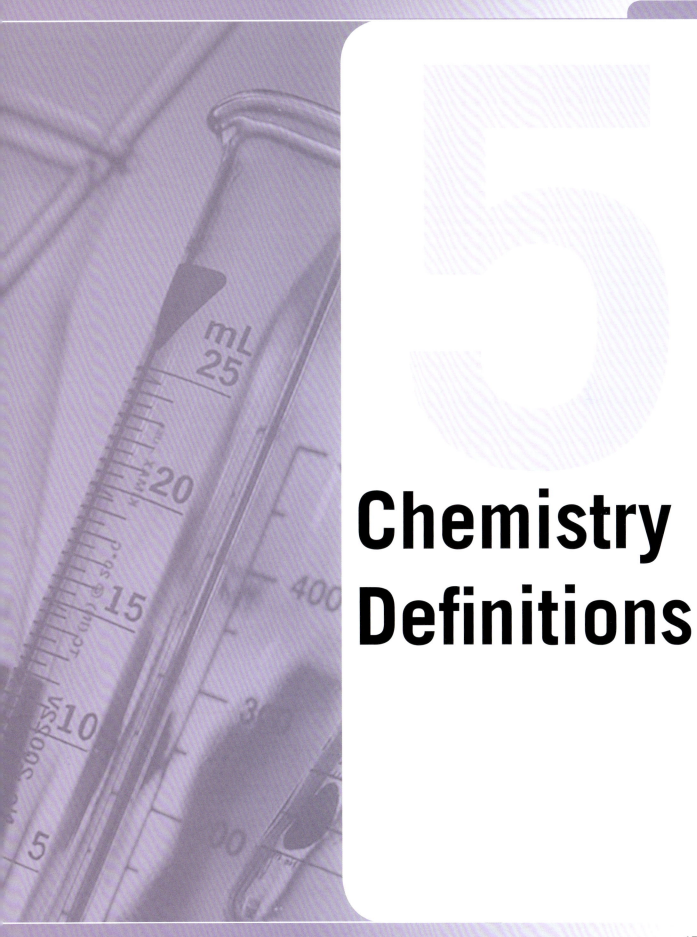

Chemistry Definitions

A

Abrasives (for topical use only):

Used to remove unwanted tissue or foreign materials from various body surfaces. The removed materials may include skin surface cells, callus, or dental plaque. As a rule, abrasives are irregularly shaped fine or coarse solids. Harder abrasives include special forms of hydrated silica used for tooth cleansing, while softer abrasives such as oatmeal are employed to remove skin surface cells that have not completed the normal desquamating process.

Absorption (skin)

A route by which substances can enter the body through the skin.

Acid:

An acid is considered any chemical compound that, when dissolved in water, gives a solution with a hydrogen ion activity greater than in pure water, i.e. a pH less than 7.0.
A substance with a pH of 0 is considered most acidic and a substance with a pH of 6.9, least acidic. Chemicals or substances having the property of an acid are said to be acidic.

Acidifying agents (acidulants):

Used in liquid preparations to provide acidic medium for product stability (e.g. lactic acid, hydrochloric acid).

Accelerator:

An accelerator is a substance that speeds up (accelerates) a chemical reaction.

Active ingredient:

The ingredient that is responsible for producing the desired effect of a mixture of ingredients and for giving the product its main characteristic. They may be proteins, vitamins, botanical extracts etc. The active ingredient is not necessarily the most common ingredient in a product.

Additives, colour (colouring agents):

Used to impart colour to liquid and solid formulations (e.g. D&C Orange #10 Lake, Flaming Red (D&C Red #36)).

Adsorbents:

Ingredients, usually solids, with a large surface area which can attract dissolved or finely dispersed substances from another medium by physical or chemical (chemisorption) means (e.g. bentonite, cellulose).

Air displacement agents:

Substances employed to displace air in a hermetically sealed container to enhance product stability (e.g. nitrogen, carbon dioxide). Used in aseptic packaging.

Alcohol:

An alcohol is any organic compound in which a hydroxyl group (-OH) is bound to a carbon atom of an alkyl or substituted alkyl group. The names of various alcohols are characterised by the suffix -ol on the end of the name. Ethanol is an example of a simple alcohol, with octyl Dodecanol an example of a fatty alcohol. Benzyl alcohol is a widely used aromatic alcohol.

Alkali:

The term alkaline describes any substance with a pH greater than 7.0. A substance with a pH of 14 is considered highly alkaline, and a pH of 7.1 minimally alkaline.

Alkalising agents:

Substances used in liquid preparations to provide alkaline medium for product stability (e.g. diethanolamine, potassium citrate)

Amino acid:

The basic building block of protein. All amino acids contain an amino (NH2) end, a carboxyl end (COOH) and a side group (R). In proteins, amino acids are joined together when the NH2 group of one forms a bond with the COOH group of the adjacent amino acid. The side group is what distinguishes each of the amino acids from the others.

Anticaking agents:

Ingredients used to prevent the agglomeration of a particulate solid into lumps or cohesive cakes. (e.g. calcium phosphate tribasic, talc).

Anticoagulants:

Substances used to prevent ingredients from changing from a fluid state to more or less solid state (e.g. edetic acid, (EDTA)).

Antifoaming agents:

Chemicals which reduce the tendency of finished products to generate foam on shaking or agitation. The ability to control foaming is important during the mixing and filling of products and in those products which should not foam during consumer use. The absence of foam provides the consumer with air-free products and facilitates maintenance of consistent fill weights during bottling.
Called antifoams for short.

Antifungal preservative:

Substance used in liquid and semi-solid preparations to prevent the growth of fungi. The effectiveness of the parabens is usually enhanced when they are used in combination (e.g. butylparaben, ethylparaben).

Antioxidant synergists:

Substances that improve the function of an antioxidant helping it to inhibit oxidation and thus is used to prevent the deterioration of preparations by the oxidative process (e.g. edetic acid (EDTA)).

Antioxidants:

Any substance that reduces oxidative damage (damage due to oxygen) such as that caused by free radicals. In formulations, can be ingredients employed to prevent or retard product spoilage from rancidity or by inhibiting oxidation (deterioration from reaction with oxygen).

Antistatic agents (for use in topically applied cosmetics):

Ingredients that alter the electrical properties of materials or of human body surfaces (skin, hair, etc.) by reducing their tendency to acquire an electrical charge.

B

Bases:

Agents used as a vehicle into which medicinal substances are incorporated (e.g. polydextrose, lanolin, hard fat).

Binders:

Ingredients added to compounded dry powder mixtures of solids and the like to provide adhesive qualities during and after compression to make tablets or cakes. Many lipids, surfactants, and polymers can be used for the indicated purpose (e.g. acacia, gelatin).

Bioactive:

Describes any material that exhibits interaction or effect on any cell tissue.

Botanical:

A constituent from a plant source that provides therapeutic or biological effect.

Buffering agents:

Chemicals which have the property of maintaining the pH of an aqueous medium in a narrow range even if small amounts of acids or bases are added. Buffering agents and pH adjusters are used to alter and to maintain a product's pH at the desired level (e.g. malic acid, sodium citrate). Called buffers for short

Bulking agents:

Usually chemically inert, solid ingredients employed as diluents for other solids. In this application bulking agents are, for example, useful in the extension of pigments for use in a powder.

C

Carrier:

A term used to describe a component of a formula that provides a number of functions including delivery of active ingredients and stability. Also known as a vehicle.

Catalyst:

A substance that speeds up a chemical reaction without being consumed itself in the reaction.

Catenation:

The bonding together of atoms of the same element to form chains. The ability of an element to bond to itself.

Cathode:

The electrode at which current flows out of a polarised electrical device.

Cation:

A positive ion; an atom or group of atoms that has lost one or more electrons.

Chain reaction:
> A reaction that, once initiated, sustains itself and expands. This is a reaction in which reactive species, such as radicals, are produced in more than one step. These reactive species, radicals, propagate the chain reaction.

Chain termination step:
> The combination of two radicals, which removes the reactive species that propagate the change reaction.

Chemical bonds:
> The attractive forces that hold atoms together in elements or compounds.

Chemical change:
> A change in which one or more new substances are formed.

Chemical equation:
> Description of a chemical reaction by placing the formulas of the reactants on the left and the formulas of products on the right of an arrow.

Chemical equilibrium:
> A state of dynamic balance in which the rates of forward and reverse reactions are equal; there is no net change in concentrations of reactants or products while a system is at equilibrium.

Chemical kinetics:
> The study of rates and mechanisms of chemical reactions and of the factors on which they depend.

Chemical periodicity:
> The variations in properties of elements with their position in the periodic table

Chelating agents:
> Ingredients that have the ability to complex with and inactivate metallic ions in order to prevent their adverse effects on the stability or appearance of products. At times it is important to complex calcium or magnesium ions which are incompatible with a variety of ingredients. Chelation of ions, such as iron or copper, helps retard oxidative deterioration of finished products (e.g. edetic acid (EDTA), maltol). Also called sequestrants.

Cis-:
> The prefix used to indicate that groups are located on the same side of a bond about which rotation is restricted.

Clarifying agent:
> Substance used as a filtering aid because of its adsorbent qualities (e.g. bentonite).

Coating agents:
> Substances used to coat a solid formulation in order to aid in stability or improve the taste or odour (e.g. sugar adjunct, cetyl alcohol).

Colouring agents (Colorant):
> Substances used to impart colour to liquid and solid (e.g. tablets and capsules) formulations (e.g. D&C Orange #10 Lake, Flaming Red (D&C Red #36)).

Colloid:
> A heterogeneous mixture in which solute-like particles do not settle out.

Combination reaction:
> Reaction in which two substances (elements or compounds) combine to form one compound. Reaction of a substance with oxygen in a highly exothermic reaction: usually shows with a visible flame.

Common ion effect:
> Suppression of ionization of a weak electrolyte by the presence in the same solution of a strong electrolyte containing one of the same ions as the weak electrolyte.

Comedogenic:
> The properties of a substance that chemically induces plugging of the pilosebaceous duct by assisting the clumping together of keratinocytes. (Hyperkeratinisation).

Complex ions:
> Ions resulting from the formation of coordinate covalent bonds between simple ions and other ions or molecules.

Compound:
> A substance of two or more elements in fixed proportions. Compounds can be decomposed into their constituent elements.

Controlled release vehicles (Extended release agents):
> Ingredients in a delivery system that allows the active component in a formulation to be released over time (e.g. microcrystalline wax, yellow wax).

Cosmeceutical:
> Cosmetic products with biologically active ingredients asserting to have medical or drug-like properties.

Covalent bond:
> Chemical bond formed by the sharing of one or more electron pairs between two atoms.

Cream:
> A semi-solid form that contains active agents dissolved or dispersed in either an oil-in-water emulsion or in another type of water-washable base.

Cream, liposomal:
> A semi-solid form that contains active agents and consists of solid particles dispersed in either an oil-in-water emulsion or in another type of water-washable base.

Cytokines:
> A large family of protein, peptide and glycoprotein signalling molecules that are secreted by certain cells of the immune system which carry signals locally between cells. Responsible for cellular communication.

D

Denaturants (for topical use only):
> Ingredients added to ethyl alcohol to make it unsuitable for product intended to be administered orally. The materials used usually have an intensely bitter taste that renders the alcohol unpalatable.

Denaturation:
> A process pertaining to changes in structure of a protein form regular to irregular arrangement of the polypeptide chains.

Density:
> Mass per unit Volume: D=MV

Delivery systems:
> Substances used to improve the delivery of the active ingredient through its route through the epidermis to its intended delivery site. (e.g. liposome).

Derivative:
> A compound that can be imagined to arise from a patent compound by replacement of one atom with another atom or group of atoms. Used extensively in organic chemistry to assist in identifying compounds.

Dermal toxicity:
> Adverse health effects resulting from skin exposure ot a substance.

Desiccants:
> Substances that trap moisture (e.g. calcium sulfate, anhydrous).

Detergents:
> Substances used to change the surface tension of a formulation to form an emulsion around certain ingredients (e.g. sodium lauryl sulfate).

Diluents:
> Substances used to dilute or reduce the concentration of the medicinal ingredient (e.g. calcium sulfate, sorbitol).

Dilution:
> The process of reducing the concentration of a solute in a solution, usually by mixing with more solvent.

Dimer:
> Molecule formed by combination of two smaller (identical) molecules.

Dipeptide
> A combination of two amino acids by means of a peptide.

Disinfectants (antimicrobial preservatives, antiseptics)
> Substances used in liquid and semi-solid preparations to prevent the growth of micro-organisms. (e.g. phenolic acid, benzalkonium chloride).

Disintegrants:

Substances used in solid dosage forms to promote the disruption of the solid mass into smaller particles which are more readily dispersed or dissolved (e.g. alginic acid, (carboxymethylcellulose).

Dispersing agents (suspending agents):

Substances that help maintain the dispersion of small particles in a formulation (e.g. poloxamer, sorbitan esters).

Displacement reactions:

Reactions in which one element displaces another from a compound.

Disproportionation reactions:

Redox reactions in which the oxidizing agent and the reducing agent are the same species.

Dissociation:

The process in which a solid ionic compound separates into its ions, in an aqueous solution.

Dissociation constant:

Equilibrium constant that applies to the dissociation of a complex ion into a simple ion and coordinating species (ligands).

Dissolution enhancing agents:

Substances that alter the molecular forces between ingredients to enhance the dissolution of the solute in the solvent (e.g. fructose, povidone).

Distilland:

The material in a distillation apparatus that is to be distilled.

Distillate:

The material in a distillation apparatus that is collected in the receiver.

Distillation:

The separation of a liquid mixture into its components on the basis of differences in boiling points. Boiling away the more volatile liquid separates the components of the mixture.

Double bond:

Covalent bond resulting from the sharing of four electrons (two pairs) between two atoms.

Dusting powders:

Powdery substances used to improve the sensory characteristics of a formulation (e.g. cornstarch, modified starch).

Dyes (colouring agents):

Substances used to impart colour to formulations (e.g. Helindone Pink (D&C Red #30), Indigotine (FD&C Blue #2).

Elastomers:

 A series of substances with rubber-like properties. Most often found in masks.

Electrolyte:

 A substance whose aqueous solutions conduct electricity.

Electrolytic cells:

 Electrochemical cells in which electrical energy causes no spontaneous redox reactions to occur. This chemical reaction occurs by the application of an outside source of electrical energy.

Electrolytic conduction:

 Conduction of electrical current by ions through a solution or pure liquid.

Electromagnetic radiation:

 Energy that is propagated by means of electric and magnetic fields that oscillates in directions perpendicular to the direction of travel of the energy.

Electron:

 A subatomic particle having a mass of 0.00054858 amu and a charge of 1-.

Electron affinity:

 The amount of energy absorbed in the process in which an electron is added to a neutral isolated gaseous atom to form a gaseous ion with a 1- charge; has a negative value if energy is released.

Electron configuration:

 Specific distribution of electrons in atomic orbitals of atoms or ions.

Electron deficient compounds:

 Compounds that contain at least one atom (other than H) that shares fewer than eight electrons

Electronic transition:

 The transfer of an electron from one energy level to another.

Element:

 A substance that cannot be decomposed into simpler substances by chemical means.

Emollients (for topical use only):

 Substances used to soften and soothe the skin (e.g. cetearyl alcohol, cholesterol).

Emulsion:

 A two-phase system that contains medicinal agents, in which one liquid is dispersed through another liquid in the form of small droplets.

Emulsifying agents:

 Substances used to promote and maintain the dispersion of finely subdivided particles of a liquid in a vehicle in which it is immiscible. The efficacy of emulsifying agents depends on their ability to reduce surface tension, to form complex films on the surface of emulsified droplets, and to create a repulsive barrier on emulsified droplets to prevent their coalescence. The end product may be a liquid emulsion or semisolid emulsion (e.g. a cream) (e.g. acacia, oleic acid).

Emulsion stabilisers:

Ingredients that assist in the formation and the stabilisation of emulsions. Emulsifying agents are required for the formation of emulsions, but their activity is materially enhanced whenever an emulsion stabiliser is included in the system. Emulsion stabilisers do not act as primary emulsifiers but prevent or reduce the coalescence of emulsified droplets by modifying the continuous or the disperse phase of the emulsion. This stabilisation may result from electrical repulsion, from changes in viscosity, or from film formation on the droplet surface (e.g. lecithin).

Emulsion stabiliser (stabilising agents):

Substances that maintain the dispersion of subdivided particles in a liquid vehicle in which it is immiscible (e.g. white wax, yellow wax).

Encapsulating agent:

Substance used to form thin shells for the purpose of enclosing a substance or formulation for ease of administration (e.g. gelatin, cellulose acetate phthalate).

Endothermic:

Describes processes that absorb heat energy.

Enzymes:

Enzymes are very efficient catalysts for biochemical reactions. They speed up reactions by providing an alternative reaction pathway of lower activation energy. Most chemical catalysts catalyse a wide range of reactions. They are not usually very selective. In contrast enzymes are usually highly selective, catalysing specific reactions only. This specificity is due to the shapes of the enzyme molecules.

Essential fatty acids (EFA's)

Key components of cellular membranes, and consequently cellular health. They are not formed by any chemical pathways within the body, and must be obtained via the diet.

Essential oil:

A concentrated, hydrophobic liquid containing volatile aroma compounds extracted from plants.

Esters:

Chemical compounds derived from the condensation of inorganic or organic acids treated with alcohols.

Exfoliants:

Mildly abrasive substances used to assist the desquamation process.

Extended release agents (controlled release agents):

Ingredients in a delivery system that allow the corrective/medicinal component in a formulation to be released over time. (e.g. carrageenan, cellulose acetate).

Exothermic:

Describes processes that release heat energy.

F

Fatty acid:

Organic acids that contain aliphatic compounds such as fats or oils.

Fillers:

Substances that allow tabletting of small amounts of medicinal ingredients to be large enough to manufacture (e.g. ethylcellulose, lactose).

Film formers:

Materials which, upon drying, produce a continuous film. These films are used for diverse purposes (e.g. gelatin, polymethacrylates).

Fixatives:

Chemicals that reduce the evaporation of fragrances or scent.

Flavonoids:

A class of plant secondary metabolites known for their antioxidant properties. Also known as Bioflavonoids.

Flow enhancers:

Substances used to improve the flow properties of a formulation (e.g. colloidal silicon dioxide).

Fragrance:

A chemical compound that has a smell or odour. Also known as an odourant.

Free radical:

Formed when oxygen atoms loose an electron and become reactive and destructive. Also known as Reactive Oxygen Species, (ROS) they are formed as a natural by-product of the normal metabolism of oxygen. The superoxide and hydroxyl radical species and are associated with cell damage.

Free radical scavengers:

More commonly known as antioxidants, they are molecules capable of slowing or preventing the oxidation of other molecules.

Formula:

Combination of symbols that indicates the chemical composition of a substance.

Formula unit:

The smallest repeating unit of a substance. The molecule for non-ionic substances

Formula weight:

The mass of one formula unit of a substance in atomic mass units.

Fragrance ingredients:

According to the International Fragrance Association, fragrance ingredients are "any basic substance used in the manufacture of fragrance materials for its odorous, odour-enhancing or blending properties". Fragrance ingredients may be obtained by chemical synthesis from synthetic, fossil, or natural raw materials, or by physical operations from natural sources. The function comprises aroma chemicals, essential oils, natural extracts, distillates and isolates, oleoresins, etc.

Ligand:

An ion, a molecule, or a molecular group that binds to another chemical entity to form a larger complex.

Liquid:

The state of matter in which a substance exhibits a characteristic readiness to flow, little or no tendency to disperse, relatively high incompressibility and, whose shape is usually determined by the container it fills. Furthermore, liquids exert pressure on the sides of a container as well as on anything within the liquid itself; this pressure is transmitted undiminished in all directions.

Lipid:

A group of naturally-occurring hydrophobic or amphiphilic molecules which includes fats, waxes, sterols and fat-soluble vitamins.

Lipophilic:

Describes a substance that dissolves in or is attracted to fats, oils or other lipids. Lipophilic functional groups or molecules prefer to be in an environment where there is no water.

Liposomes:

In essence formulations utilising liposomes are a specialised polyphase, or W/OW emulsion. Where phospholipids represent a major part of the oil phase. The liposomal structure allows slow osmotic diffusion of water or water-soluble agents through the lipid membrane and into lowers layers of the epidermis.

Lotion:

A broad term to describe a liquid or semi-liquid preparation that contains cosmetic/corrective or medicinal agents, with solid materials suspended in an aqueous vehicle. Lotions are usually a suspension of solids in an aqueous medium, but may also be emulsions or solutions.

Lubricants:

Substances that reduce or prevent friction.

M

Mass:

A measure of the amount of matter in an object. Mass is usually measured in grams or kilograms.

Matter:

Anything that has mass and occupies space.

Mechanism:

The sequence of steps by which reactants are converted into products.

Melting point:

The temperature at which liquid and solid coexist in equilibrium; also the freezing point.

Miscibility:

The ability of one liquid to mix with (dissolve in) another liquid.

Mixture:

A sample of matter composed of two or more substances, each of which retains its identity and properties.

Mole:

The mole is defined as the amount of substance of a system that contains as many "elemental entities" (e.g. atoms, molecules, ions, electrons) as there are atoms in 12 g of carbon-12.

Molality:

Concentration expressed as number of moles of solute per kilogram of solvent.

Molar solubility:

Number of moles of a solute that dissolve to produce a litre of saturated solution.

Molecular equation:

Equation for a chemical reaction in which all formulas are written as if all substances existed as molecules; only complete formulas are used.

Molecular formula:

Formula that indicates the actual number of atoms present in a molecule of a molecular substance.

Molecular weight:

The mass of one molecule of a non-ionic substance in atomic mass units.

Molecule:

The smallest particle of an element or compound capable of a stable, independent existence formed from a group of a minimum of two atoms in a fixed arrangement held together by very strong chemical (covalent) bonds.

Mousse:

A foamy preparation applied externally in a pressurized container

Multiple emulsions:

This development in cosmetic chemistry is better known as a controlled release delivery system, and up until recently has been used mostly in the field of pharmacy because of difficulty in stability and extended shelf life. As the name suggests this type of formulation delivers its active ingredients over a longer time frame than would a water or oil based formula.

Nanosome:

Nanosomes (or nanoparticles) are very small, single or double bilayer Liposomes that are so small they are measured in the Nanometer range.

Natural moisturising factor:

Also known as the NMF, it is a fluid composed of water-soluble compounds including amino acids found in the stratum corneum (top layer) of the skin.

Neutralisation:

A process occurring when the excess acid (or excess base) in a substance is reacted with added base (or added acid) so that the resulting substance is neither acidic nor basic. In theory neutralization involves adding acid or base as required to achieve pH 7.

Nucleons:

Particles comprising the nucleus; protons and neutrons.

Nucleus:

The very small, very dense, positively charged centre of an atom containing protons and neutrons, as well as other subatomic particles.

Nuclides:

A specific type of atom that is characterized by its nuclear properties, such as the number of neutrons and protons and the energy state of its nucleus

Non-ionic surfactants:

Substances that absorb to surfaces or interfaces to reduce surface or interfacial tension (e.g. docusate sodium, cetrimide).

Occlusion:

In cosmetics this usually refers to a shield or film that is spread onto the skin to slow or prevent moisture evaporation. This shield or film is usually made up of materials, such as oils and waxes that cannot be penetrated by water.

Ointment bases:

Semisolid vehicle into which drug substances may be incorporated in preparing medicated ointments (e.g. lanolin alcohol, petrolatum).

Oil:

A liquid preparation consisting of an oil phase dispersed throughout an aqueous phase in such a manner that liposomes are formed. (A liquid tri-ester of glycerol and unsaturated fatty acids).

Oil-in-water (O/W) emulsion:

These formulas are water based with a small quantity of oil-based ingredients. Logically, O/W formulations will have higher moisturising and hydrating properties and be absorbed into the skin more readily than W/O emulsions. (O/W= small amount of oil into large amount of water)

Oil free emulsions:

These formulations contain no oils" but may contain modern ingredients that impart oil-like properties, such as silicones and modified lipids. This group of formulas are usually alcohol or water based lipids or a gel-like substance.

Oleaginous vehicles:

A carrying agent for a medicinal ingredient with oily properties (e.g. canola oil, cottonseed oil).

Opacifying agents:

Ingredients deliberately added to products to reduce their clear or transparent appearance.
Some opacifying agents provide the pearly appearance desired in certain products. Other opacifying agents are used for covering purposes and to hide blemishes. Most emulsions and suspensions are opaque as a result of the presence of a liquid or solid disperse phase.
Thus, a very large number of substances could be classified as opacifying agents.

Organic chemistry:

The chemistry of substances that contain carbon-hydrogen bonds.

Osmosis:

The process by which solvent molecules pass through a semipermeable membrane from a dilute solution into a more concentrated solution.

Osmotic pressure:

The hydrostatic pressure produced on the surface of a semipermable membrane by osmosis.

Oxide:

A binary compound of oxygen.

Oxidising agents:

Chemicals which gain electrons during their reaction with a reducing agent. Oxidising agents commonly contribute oxygen to other substances.

Oxidation:

Algebraic increases in the oxidation number; may correspond to a loss of electrons.

Oxidation-reduction reactions:

Reactions in which oxidation and reduction occur; also called redox reactions.

P

Parabens:

A class of chemicals widely used as preservatives in the cosmetic and pharmaceutical industries. For use in cosmetics, they are synthetically produced, although some are identical to those found in nature.

Penetrants, skin (skin penetrants) (for use in topically applied cosmetics):

Substances that promote the passage of the cosmetic/active or medicinal ingredient into the skin (e.g. alcohol, oleic acid)

Penetration enhancing agents (for use in topically applied cosmetics):

Substances that promote the passage of the cosmetic active or medicinal ingredient through its route of administration (e.g. isopropyl myristate).

Peptides:

Short polymers formed from the linking (in a defined order) of alpha-amino acids. The link between one amino acid residue and the next is called an amide bond or peptide bond.

Periodicity:

Regular periodic variations of properties of elements with atomic number (and position in the periodic table).

Periodic law:

The properties of the elements are periodic functions of their atomic numbers.

Periodic table:

An arrangement of elements in order of increasing atomic numbers that also emphasizes periodicity.

pH:

The pH scale is used to measure the acidity or alkalinity of substances. The scale is 0-14, with 7.0 being neutral. (Neither acidic or alkaline) The scale is logarithmic, so pH 4 is ten times as acidic as pH 5 and pH 3 is hundred times as acidic as pH 5, and so on.

pH adjusters:

Chemicals (acids, bases, or buffering agents) which are used to control the pH of finished products.

Photon:

A packet of light or electromagnetic radiation; also called quantum of light

Pigments (colouring agents):

Substances used to impart colour to liquid and solid formulations (e.g. titanium dioxide).

Plasticisers:

Materials which soften synthetic polymers. They are frequently required to avoid brittleness and cracking of film formers. Water, sometimes in combination with hygroscopic materials, is the common plasticizer for natural polymers and proteins. A variety of organic substances, such as esters, have been found useful for plasticizing synthetic polymers (e.g. lanolin alcohols, mineral oil).

Polymer:

Polymers are large molecules that are made up of many units (monomers) linked together in a chain. There are naturally occurring polymers (eg, starch and DNA) and synthetic polymers (eg, nylon and silicone).

Polyphenols:

A group of chemical substances found in plants that exhibit antioxidant properties with potential health benefits.

Precursors:

Compounds that participate in the chemical reactions that produces other compounds.

Potential energy:

Energy that matter possesses by virtue of its position, condition or composition.

Precipitate:

An insoluble solid formed by mixing in solution the constituent ions of a slightly soluble solution.

Primary Standard:

A substance of a known high degree of purity that undergoes one invariable reaction with the other reactant of interest.

Preservatives, antimicrobial (Antimicrobial preservatives):

Ingredients which prevent or retard microbial growth and thus protect products from spoilage (e.g. benzoic acid, benzyl alcohol). The use of preservatives is required to prevent product damage caused by microorganisms and to protect the product from inadvertent contamination by the consumer during use. The use of more than one preservative can sometimes increase efficacy due to synergism. Ingredients used to protect products against oxidative damage are classified as antioxidants.

Propellants:

Chemicals used for expelling products from pressurized containers (aerosols). The functionality of a propellant depends on its vapour pressure at ambient temperature and its compressibility. Liquids or gases can be used as propellants as long as the pressure developed within the container is safely below the container's bursting pressure under normal storage and use conditions.

Protectants:

Substances that provide a physical protection from the effects of the active ingredient (e.g. petrolatum).

Protein:

Organic compounds comprised of amino acids arranged in a linear chain and folded into a globular form. The amino acids in the chain are joined together by peptide bonds.

Proton:

A proton is a positively charge particle that resides within the atomic nucleus. The number of protons in the atomic nucleus is what determines the atomic number, as outlined in the periodic table of elements.

R

Radical:

An atom or group of atoms that contains one or more unpaired electrons (usually very reactive species) Also known as Free Radicals and Reactive Oxygen Species.

Retinoids:

A class of chemical compounds related chemically to vitamin A. Used in skin care formulations for their properties in regulating epithelial cell growth.

Reactants:

Substances consumed in a chemical reaction.

Reactive oxygen species (ROS)

Free radicals that contain the oxygen atom.

Reagents:

Chemicals that react or participate in a reaction. Some examples are solvents and oxidisers.

Reducing agent:

The substance that reduces another substance and is oxidized.

Supersaturated solution:

A solution that contains a higher than saturation concentration of solute; slight disturbance or seeding causes crystallisation of excess solute.

Surface modifiers:

Substances that may be added to other ingredients to make them more hydrophilic or hydrophobic. As a rule, surface modifiers form a covalent bond with the substrate.

Surface tension:

The cohesive forces between liquid molecules are responsible for the phenomenon known as surface tension. The molecules at the surface do not have other "like" molecules on all sides of them and consequently they cohere more strongly to those directly associated with them on the surface. This forms a surface "film "which makes it more difficult to move an object through the surface than to move it when it is completely submersed.

Surfactants:

Substances that absorb to surfaces or interfaces to reduce surface or interfacial tension. May be used as cleansing agents, hydrotropes, or emulsifying agents (e.g. docusate sodium, cetrimide).

Surfactants - cleansing agents:

Surfactants used for skin and cleaning purposes and as emulsifiers. In this function, surfactants wet body surfaces, emulsify or solubilise oils, and suspend soil.

Surfactants - foam boosters:

Surfactants used to increase the foaming capacity of Surfactants - Cleansing agents, or to stabilize foams in general. Foam boosters are substances which increase the surface viscosity of the liquid which surrounds the individual bubbles in a foam.

Surfactants - hydrotropes:

Surfactants which have the ability to enhance the water solubility of another surfactant. Prominent members of this group are short chain alkyl aryl sulfonates, sulfosuccinates, and some non-ionic surfactants.

Surfactants - solubilising agents:

Surfactants which aid in the dissolution of an ingredient (solute) in a medium in which it is not otherwise soluble. This definition is specific and excludes cosolvency, i.e., the use of a mixed solvent such as alcohols and water in a clear fragrance product. It also excludes changes in solubility affected by pH modification, such as the dissolution of lauric acid in aqueous ammonium hydroxide.

Surfactants - suspending agents:

Substances used to help distribute an insoluble solid in a liquid phase. Suspensions or dispersions of liquids in a second liquid are generally called emulsions.

Superoxide anion

A harmful derivative of oxygen capable of oxidative destruction of cell components. Free radical created by UV light.

Suspending agents (dispersing agents) - non-surfactant:

A group of ingredients which facilitate the dispersion of solids in liquids. They function primarily by coating the solid through the process of adsorption, thus changing the surface characteristic of the suspended solid.

Suspension:

A liquid pharmaceutical form that contains medicinal agents and consists of solid particles dispersed through a liquid phase in which the particles are not soluble.

Suspension, liposomal:

A liquid preparation consisting of an oil phase dispersed throughout an aqueous phase in such a manner that liposomes are formed.

Sustained release ingredients (extended-release ingredients):

Ingredients in a delivery system that allow the medicinal component in a formulation to be released over time. (e.g. carrageenan, cellulose acetate).

Texturisers:

Substances used to maintain a given viscosity, texture or control the melting point of a formulation. (Also known as stabilisers).

Thickening agents:

Substances used to change the consistency of a preparation to render it more resistant to flow (e.g. hydroxypropyl cellulose, polyethylene oxide).

Ultra Violet Radiation

Infrared (IR) visible (VIS) and Ultra Violet Radiation (UVR) are among the total spectrum of radiation that the sun emits: these three command most of our attention. UVR is of most relevance when looking at sunscreen formulations. The UV portion covers 200nm to 400nm. UVR is in turn, divided into UVC (200nm to 290nm), UVB (290nm to 320nm) and UVA (320nm to 400nm).

Unsaturated hydrocarbons:

Hydrocarbons that contain double or triple carbon-carbon bonds. Amino Acids

UVC (200nm to 290nm)

UVC is very toxic, it is lethal to many micro-organisms, such as bacteria, yeast's and protozoa, as well also to most plant life and in addition are carcinogenic to humans. Fortunately, virtually all UVC is filtered out by the ozone layer, but we know that this is gradually changing around the world.

UVA (320nm to 400nm)

Recent studies have definitively established that the longer UVA is a causative factor in photo ageing. It is also the portion of the UVR spectrum most often associated with photosensitivity's resulting from drugs or disease. UVA also penetrates the skin to a greater depth than UVB. UVA is also further divided into UVA II & I (340-400 nm) (320-340 nm). Referred to as long and short UVA respectively. The relatively large amount of UVA and its ability to penetrate deeply into the skin (dermal layer) accounts for its greater significance when establishing cause of skin ageing.

UVB (290nm to 320nm)

Most of this UVB is filtered out by the atmosphere, and makes up approximately 1% of the UVR that reaches the e arth's surface. However, despite its relatively low presence, UVB is associated with much of the damage caused to humans by sun exposure. UVB has been credited as being the sole cause of sunburn and various skin cancers. It is 100 times more time more efficient in producing erythema than UVA.

V-Z

Viscosity-decreasing agents:

Substance used to enhance the fluidity of products without a significant lowering of the concentration of the active constituents. Inorganic salts, organic salts, solvents, and a few selected substances have the ability to lower the viscosity of products. Their efficacy depends on their concentration and is highly specific for each type of product.

Viscosity-increasing agents:

Substances used to change the consistency of a preparation to render it more resistant to flow. Used in suspensions to deter sedimentation, in ophthalmic solutions to enhance contact time or to thicken topical creams (e.g. cetearyl alcohol, sodium alginate).

Viscosity-increasing agents - aqueous:

Substances used to thicken the aqueous portions of products. Their ability to perform this function is related to their water solubility or hydrophilic nature.

Viscosity-increasing agents - non-aqueous:

Substances used to thicken the lipid portions of products. Their performance is the result of their water insolubility and compatibility with various lipids. They are widely used to thicken or gel various types of oleaginous products.

Vitamins, stabilising agents for:

A substance that helps to prevent deterioration of a vitamin, thus maintaining stability (e.g. propylene glycol).

Water-absorbing agents:

Substances that can hold water, thereby altering the thickness of a formulation (e.g. carboxymethyl-cellulose calcium).

Water in oil (W/O):

Small amount of water into a large amount of oil. Used to be known as night creams. Occlusive action that slows evaporation of water from the Stratum Corneum, and temporaily restores the acid mantle.

Water-miscible cosolvents:

A solvent that is able to mix with water (e.g. edetic acid (EDTA)).

Wetting agents:

A substance, usually a surface-active agent, which reduces the surface tension of a liquid and therefore increases its adhesion to a solid surface (e.g. benzalkonium chloride, poloxamer).

Regulatory bodies & associations of interest

International Federation of Societies of Cosmetic Chemists (International)
The IFSCC is a worldwide federation dedicated to international cooperation in cosmetic science and technology
www.ifscc.org

The Australian society of Cosmetic Chemists
The Australian Society of Cosmetic Chemists is a professional scientific organisation that promotes the advancement of the theory and practice of the science and technology of cosmetics, toiletries and perfumery. Membership is open to individuals who are working or interested in the cosmetics, toiletries and perfumery industry. *www.ascc.com.au*

TGA (Australia)
The TGA assesses cosmetic products that make therapeutic claims. Many ingredients in cosmetic products are classed as industrial chemicals and the National Industrial Chemicals Notification Assessment Scheme (NICNAS) must be notified of all cosmetics that contain industrial chemicals new to Australia. *www.tga.govt.au*

International Fragrance Association (International)
IFRA represents the fragrance industry and national associations worldwide. Research and development, scientific findings, health and safety concerns as well as environmental protection are at the heart of IFRA's concerns. Together with the industry's scientific arm the Research Institute for Fragrance Materials (RIFM), IFRA ensures that the establishment of usage Standards for fragrance materials are put into practice according to available scientific recommendations, and that all member companies comply with those Standards. Self-regulation enables the IFRA Standards to be adopted very rapidly by fragrance houses worldwide and by the industry as a whole.
www.ifraorg.org

FDA (United States)
The Food and Drug Administration (FDA or USFDA) is a Government agency of the United States Department of Health and Human Services and is responsible for regulating and supervising the safety of foods, tobacco products, dietary supplements, Medication drugs, vaccines, Biopharmaceutical, blood transfusion, medical devices, Electromagnetic radiation emitting devices, veterinary products, and cosmetics.
www.fda.gov

Cosmetic Toiletry and Fragrance Association of NZ
The association was formed in 1972 by a core group of companies who were manufacturing most of their products in New Zealand at the time. Prime objectives then were to present a united front and to lobby government in the interests of member companies. While these objectives remain, the restructuring of the New Zealand economy over the past two decades has seen an expanded focus by the CTFA. Our industry has changed dramatically. Today, worldwide consolidation has meant much of New Zealand's requirements are imported. Company mergers and acquisitions have altered the landscape, while niche marketing and contract manufacturing have also contributed to the change. Issues like HSNO, parallel importing, regulation and harmonisation, along with government bureaucracy, will have considerable influence on the future direction of our industry. The CTFA will play a major role in determining that direction.
www.ctfa.org.nz

Personal Care Products Council (United States)
The Personal Care Products Council (formerly the Cosmetic, Toiletry and Fragrance Association) is the leading national trade association for the cosmetic and personal care products industry and represents the most innovative names in beauty today. For more than 600 member companies, they are the voice on scientific, legal, regulatory, legislative and international issues for the personal care product industry. They are a leading and trusted source of information for and about the industry and a vocal advocate for consumer safety and continued access to new, innovative products. *www.personalcarecouncil.org*

Colipa (Europe)
Colipa represents the interests of more than 2000 companies ranging from major international cosmetics manufacturers to small family-run businesses operating in niche markets. Together, these employ more than 500,000 people within the European Union.
The products that come within the scope of Colipa extend across a divers range that includes essential personal hygiene products such as deodorant, shampoo and toothpaste as well as beauty preparations.
More than 5 billion personal hygiene items are sold every year. Virtually everyone in Europe uses at least one product every day, soap for example. Decisions to buy and use of cosmetics are closely linked to lifestyle, and this makes research and development vital to the cosmetics industry as manufacturers respond to increasingly sophisticated consumer demand.
Colipa's members are committed to continuing development of safe, innovative and effective products.
Their mission is to meet consumer desires for new and enhanced products and to provide useful and more comprehensive product information. *www.colipa.eu/about-colipa.html*